PROSTRANAL

The Ultimate Guide to Prostate Orgasms

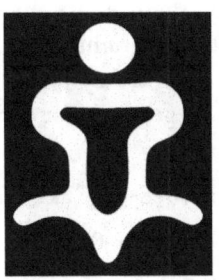

ERIC WIN

ISBN (Hardcover): ISBN: 979-8-9928772-1-2

ISBN (Paperback): 979-8-9928772-0-5

ISBN (eBook): 979-8-9928772-2-9

prostranal.com

Published by

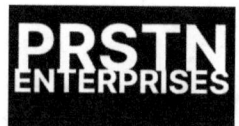

CONTENTS

I dedicate this book to my late father and to my wife, whose unwavering support and encouragement made this journey possible. A special thanks to everyone I've met in the sexual wellness community, whose passion and insights continue to inspire me—I honor you for shaping the industry and working to make the world a better place.

PREFACE

If you're a dedicated student, you could be experiencing anal orgasms within 30 days.

Congratulations on taking the first step! If you can get over the social stigma of putting something in your anus, you're on the path to unlimited pleasure. Just know that this journey takes time to get the hang of it, and your utmost patience is required.

Exploring this new world will be half the fun. And it is more mental than physical. **Don't expect prostate orgasms to be anything like the penile orgasms you are used to having**—they will be much better once you have your first breakthrough!

My first encounter with multiple orgasms occurred in my twenties. I was dating a woman who could have several orgasms (back-to-back, every 30-60 seconds) during sex. It left me in awe. And I became envious of the female vagina after those months with her. I thought having a cock was the ultimate source of pleasure, but watching her yoni gush fluids, and endlessly contract, for an hour or more made me question the quality of my own, boring penile orgasms. So, I spent the next few decades chasing multi-orgasmic lovers—let's just say, women like that aren't easy to find.

The next chapters of my life brought me to a search for the holy grail of anal orgasms. I came across a forum post in my early forties that evolved into a discussion about prostate orgasms. Several men chimed in, proclaiming anal orgasms to be the ultimate experience. But they vaguely mentioned what they were doing, or how they were going about it. This captured my interest and led me to explore deeper. I went searching the internet to see what else was out there on the topic.

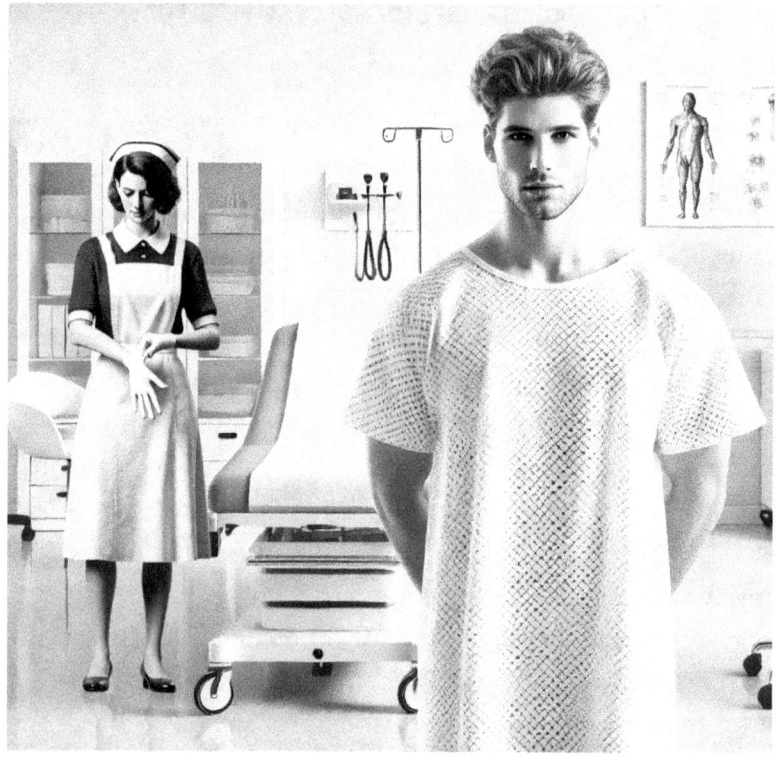

After reading this book, a scene like this take on a whole new meaning.

I'd seen the movie *Road Trip* (2000) and remembered the famed E.L. (Seann William Scott) prostate scene, where he ejaculates when the nurse inserts her fingers in his rectum and manipulates his prostate—the nurse describes this as "milking the prostate". I'd always thought it was an urban legend. I began to doubt the truth of these internet posters, thinking they were just trolling expeditions. But when I discovered a few prostate orgasm forums, I soon realized there was a whole new world lurking beneath the surface of traditional men's orgasms. A thriving community of "prostrainers" existed. And I was determined to uncover their secrets!

The greatest challenge for me was figuring out where to start. I was familiar with the feeling of having a finger (hers or mine) inserted in my rectum during sex or masturbation and how it enhanced orgasms. But I had no clue how to make a prostate orgasm happen. The posts on these sites were fragmented, with no structure. There were more questions than answers.

One internet poster mentioned a Hitachi wand with an attachment. He went into some detail about how good it felt. Intrigued, I bought one online; however, it was not the right "fit". After that, I bought another attachment that was marketed for "Anal P-Gasms" and advertised as "ergonomically better". I remember just sitting there for five minutes, not sure of what I was supposed to feel. I didn't notice anything particularly stimulating, and I quickly became bored.

A few weeks later I tried again. This time I could feel some light, electrical sensations, but nothing significant. I also tried a couple other toys and methods. Mostly though, I would masturbate by hand and cum with a plug or toy inside me. This felt amazing! It led me to experiment with getting close to climax, then stopping and pushing the plug in and out, or squeezing on it with my sphincter muscles and holding down for as long as I could. I'd edge for an hour doing this. At times, it felt like I was going to cum hands-free. Little did I know, but I was gradually moving from less penis play into more ass play, associating pleasure with the prostate.

This was the start of the awakening inside my body. But all the while, I still doubted I'd ever have the sensational anal orgasms that I was reading about online (i.e., cumming hands-free or having 10-30 minutes of nonstop orgasms). My progress was slow and sometimes it felt like I was going backward.

But quitters never prosper—or prostate! I refused to give up on this journey. And after a few months of trying daily, I finally experienced my first set of P-Waves from my Hitachi toy setup. A P-Wave is a profound sensation of euphoria originating from the lower abdomen or pelvic area, distinct from genital stimulation—think of it like tremors before the earthquake.

A few days later, I had my first round of hands-free, dry anal orgasms. Of course, this became addictive, but not fully satisfying. I wanted more pleasure and knew there was more to come (pun intended). I discovered hands-free orgasm videos online and was inspired to continue experimenting. This benchmark became my obsession and ultimate goal.

Fast forward . . . it took me over a year to finally experience a ferocious hands-free wet orgasm. Thereafter, I thoroughly dedicated myself to the practice. It changed my entire approach to sex and pleasure.

I wrote this book because I was frustrated with the shortage of answers and clear information online. **Prostate education should be accessible to all, as the value of learning prostate-play is simply too good to ignore.** No one had produced a comprehensive manual to make it easy for men to achieve anal orgasms. And there is no reason that only cisgender women should have multiple, explosive orgasms.

Penis-owner anatomy is also designed to experience this kind of pleasure.

This is the perfect opportunity for new thrills and unforgettable experiences! Whether you're an adventurous spirit eager to discover a unique kind of delight, or even if you're typically more reserved, this enticing experience promises something special that you have been missing out on.

So let's get started on your voyage. It's time to explore your centers of joy and transform your pleasure pathways to experience an exhilarating journey of discovery!

Live Long and Prostate!

Eric Win
"The Prostate Prophet"

Visit **prostranal.com** for more information, advanced training, and the latest resources.

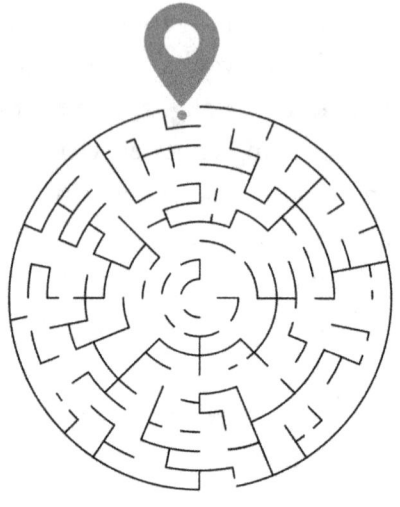

You're at the entrance of the maze. I'll walk you through the next few chapters. We'll cover key terms, arousal techniques, anatomy, and everything you need to unlock an anal orgasm. Trust me, it's worth it. And don't worry—the fun part is coming soon (pun intended).

DISCLAIMER

The information provided in this book is for entertainment and informational purposes only and should not be taken as medical advice. I am not a scientist or a doctor. This book is a quasi-anatomy, Tantra, self-help, coaching sex manual that is not looking to be peer-reviewed scientifically or held up foundationally in the medical community.

The information contained herein should not be used in place of, or as a substitute for, the advice of an appropriately qualified and licensed physician or other healthcare provider. The user of this information is solely responsible for determining whether the information contained herein is appropriate for the user's intended use and should consult a qualified healthcare provider before taking any action based on this information.

This information is provided "as is" without warranty of any kind, either express or implied, including but not limited to: the implied warranties of merchantability, fitness for a particular purpose, or non-infringement. The information contained herein is subject to change and does not represent a commitment on the part of the author and/or publisher.

Any trademark products mentioned in this book are owned by their respective companies and are used for descriptive purposes only, with no claim to endorsement or affiliation with the trademark owner(s). Any trademarked product does not originate, and is not sourced from, this work and stands independently to the author with no representation intended.

The author and publisher expressly disclaim any and all liability arising directly or indirectly from the use of, or reliance upon, the information contained herein. The user of this information assumes all risks from the use or misuse of the information contained herein, including any injury, loss, or damage incurred as a result of such use or misuse.

The precision and veracity of events recounted herein are subject to significant limitations in recall and accuracy. Said limitations stem from the inherent fallibility of the author's memory concerning the sequence, detail, and factual integrity of the occurrences as described. Consequently, the reader should consider that the recounting of events, while undertaken in good faith, may not comprehensively or accurately reflect the exactitude of the historical or factual circumstances. It is expressly acknowledged by the author that the recollection of events may be, at best, a partial and imprecise representation of reality. Reader discretion is advised.

By using this information, the reader agrees to indemnify and hold harmless the author and publisher from and against any and all claims, damages, costs, and expenses arising from the use of or reliance upon the information contained herein.

In short, seek medical consultation before exploring your ass and urogenital region.

*NOTE: This book is perfect for all genders to enjoy reading; however, is not intended for cis women born with vaginas since it focuses on the prostate and associated pathways—**it is intended for those born with a penis and a prostate**. Nevertheless, all women are encouraged to use this book in conjunction with their partners as it can help enhance sexual pleasure and wellness e.g., introducing pegging, exploring giving multiple orgasms, etc. That said, some of the arousal amplification techniques in this book are universal and can be applied to those (without a prostate) seeking to have anal orgasms from intercourse or manual stimulation.*

FOREWORD

With *Prostranal*, Eric Win boldly goes where no author has gone before—the prostate's role in sexual pleasure. For most men, the prostate is a bystander. How can you make it a player on stage, or maybe take the lead? This book will reward you with ideas and techniques that most have not considered. You will be enlightened about a taboo subject. And his style is charming, candid, and clear.

First, what qualifies me as an expert reviewer? I am Elliot Justin, MD, founder of FirmTech, the leader in sextech wearables for better sexual health and heightened performance and pleasure. Second, like Eric I have been very open minded since I could first get an erection about self-experimentation on any reasonable (and some less so) tool, technique or substance that might make sex better for myself and my lovers. Before we recommend anything, we first trial it on ourselves.

In the twenty-first century, we are enjoying a wave of sexual breakthroughs that are providing objective, actionable and personal benefits that are prolonging our years of lovemaking and popularizing fresh pleasures and intimacies. What were regarded as fetish and edgy are now enjoyed by many. Vibrators are mainstream; they left the bottom drawer at the turn of the century. Cock rings are coming out of the closet. Role play? If you aren't doing it, you are imagining it. Admit it!

Doctors know that the prostate gland produces ejaculate fluid. Equally significant, it converts testosterone to biologically active dihydrotestosterone (DHT). Eric's focus is different and more compelling for mankind. He is the pioneer of the prostate, exploring its objective and subjective role in sexual pleasure. In *Prostranal*, we learn about his explorations of its powerful role in pleasure.

Prostate pleasure is real and can be enjoyed by men who are open minded. If you've never tried prostate sex—you're not alone. That's rapidly changing. Increasingly, straight men as well as gay men are making it a regular part of their sexual play.

Prostranal offers innovative techniques and powerful story-telling to help rewire your body's pleasure systems and unlock intense edging and climaxes. Eric is bold, honest and inclusive. He gives men tools and advice that will inspire and help them to discover how prostate stimulation will be a game changer for them solo and with partners emotionally and physically.

Thank you, Eric! Men and their doctors are a long way from frank discussions about prostate and anal sex. Your book works as a guide and confidant in this still taboo area.

Sexual pleasure and lovemaking of course have subjective and objective parts. As a doctor, I am interested in both. Men like Eric can testify to the subjective side. I am also intrigued by the objective side. Can we quantify the benefits? Does prostate stimulation increase blood flow? Does it increase PC (pubococcygeus) muscle contractions that occur during orgasms? Can regular prostate sex address low testosterone and erectile dysfunction? Do pelvic floor exercises heighten prostate sensitivity and/or increase penile blood flow?

Eric Win's *Prostranal* welcomes the adventurous, the curious, and the cautious. It's time for you to explore and enjoy the frontier of prostate sex.

Elliot Justin, MD, RingMaster

CHAPTER 1

JUST THE TIP: AN INTRODUCTION

Overview

This is where I try to convince you that doing this is a good idea. I'll kick things off with my first vulnerable story, hoping you'll stick around for five more chapters. And honestly, I'm grinning just thinking about your priceless facial expressions when you get to the stories at the end of the book —especially the shower scene.

Our bodies are unique. And just like cars, they come with their own settings and configurations. Unfortunately, we were not given an instruction manual or navigation system for experiencing pleasure. This guide is the next best thing to help you unlock the power of prostate play.

If you want to uncover the secrets of anal pleasure, all you have to do is "interrogate" the prostate until it reveals the answers. But first, **you need to decipher and learn the language of your body**. Exploring it is a delightful journey not limited to any particular gender or sexual orientation. It can bring immense pleasure when located and manipulated correctly. As you explore, you will discover that you do not need to use only your penis to achieve multiple orgasms. **Your prostate is wanting to be milked**, it is quietly screaming, "Your anus is a gateway to infinite pleasure!"

> In some cultures, the prostate is known as "the second heart". Anatomically, it is the heart of the reproductive system.

But remember, sex is complicated, and everything connects to your sexual state of being. The pieces of the puzzle include your physical, mental, and emotional state. To experience anal bliss, you must connect these three together. And since not all bodies work the same, **anal pleasure starts as a journey of self-discovery.** The key is to not worry about when the orgasm will happen or seek a specific outcome. Instead, have fun while safely exploring your body.

In your own time, you will discover what works for you. And know that this practice will take dedicated time. Learning to relax and slow down comprises a big part of the process. You have to train through trial and error, learning what feels good to your mind and body. This book provides you with proven arousal amplification techniques while offering encouragement along the way.

Your curiosity brought you this far . . . and you are not alone! The increasing demand for anal toys, and the growing interest in prostate pleasure continues to rise. These sales are not solely driven by gay and queer consumers. In fact, our society has long associated anal play and prostate pleasure with gay and bisexual men, despite the fact that not all men who have sex with men engage in anal play.

Unfortunately, this absurd association is often the fuel for homophobia, which stereotypes any straight man who enjoys anal stimulation as weak or freaky. As a result, **many men may feel hesitant or ashamed to explore their bodies and embrace the pleasure that prostate stimulation brings to everyone on the sexual spectrum.**

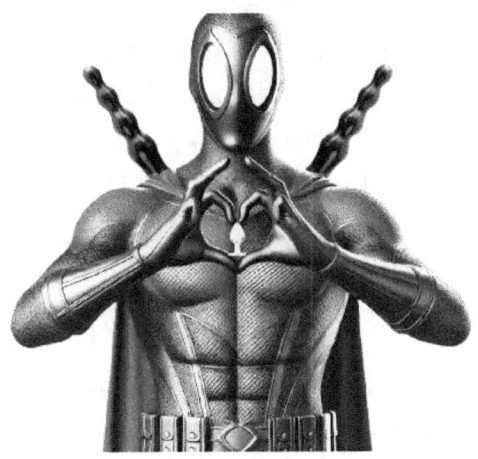

Deadpool's long-lost brother, Buttpool, knows that butt stuff is good stuff.

I encourage you to focus on the pleasure—not the labels. Remember, being straight and exploring your prostate will not "turn you gay". Just as putting your dick into a vagina doesn't make you straight.

Personal Story: I remember one time masturbating in my adolescence. Somehow I decided to insert a finger in my ass just before climaxing. The feeling of shame and guilt afterward stayed with me for weeks. I would finger myself off and on over the years, and I felt terrible each time. I never had sexual feelings for men or even "gay thoughts". Despite the negative emotions, it felt so good that I could not stop enjoying this sensation from time to time.

In college, I finally felt vindicated when a girlfriend asked if she could put a finger inside me during sex. Elated and pretending to be innocent, I happily agreed. After several more girlfriends, it was hit-and-miss finding women who would tickle my prostate with their finger. Fortunately, with age it became easier. I've discovered a vibrant world of open-minded women, eager to connect with men who enjoy prostate play, and will gladly reverse roles in the bedroom.

Nowadays, **you see the topic of anal play trending in mainstream comedy, movies, and songs more and more**. Just do a search on IMDB (e.g., **imdb.com/search/title/?keywords=pegging**) to see the rising popularity. As a result, the rising demand for prostate toys is likely a reflection of the growing visibility and acceptance of all forms of sexuality in our culture. More people are rejecting outdated societal norms and "loosening up". They are starting to see that anal stimulation has no boundaries.

It is time to continue to break down the remaining barriers and stigma surrounding this type of pleasure and recognize that it is a healthy part of human sexuality. By doing so, we can empower individuals of all genders and sexual orientations to explore their bodies, discover new sensations, and embrace their sexuality without shame or fear of judgment. **A prostate orgasm is truly a mind-shattering event and nothing like any other orgasm you've ever experienced.** I predict that anal orgasms will be the new norm for heterosexual men in the next 20 years once more people embrace this knowledge.

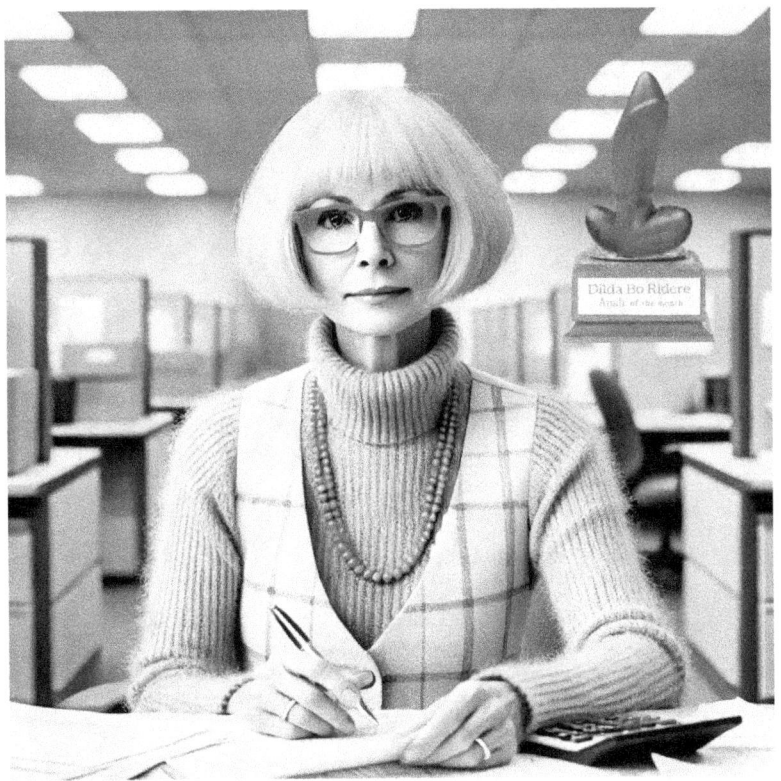

Diedre Beaubeirdre's cousin, Dilda Bo Ridere, is waiting for the green light on a sequel titled Everything Everywhere All Inside At Once.

CHAPTER 2

DECODING ANAL ORGASMS

Overview

- Learn key terms and types of orgasms related to prostate play.
- Explore different orgasmic experiences and their variations.
- There's a lot to take in, but don't stress—I'll break it down at the end of the chapter to keep it simple.

The prostate, also sometimes referred to as the "male G-Spot" or P-Spot, is part of the reproductive system and located within the urogenital system. This gland is surrounded by numerous nerves and vessels. They connect to the autonomic nervous system through many inner organs, and to the brain through blood hormones released by the testes and the pituitary gland. Controlling the flow of semen and urine, it acts like a traffic light controller for the urethra by managing the stream of different fluids depending on the body's needs.

From a Tantra standpoint, **the prostate acts as the emotional center**, also referred to by certain enlightened people as the "sacred spot". For many individuals, an emotional outpouring occurs when having a prostate orgasm.

Let's explore the types and terms associated with prostate play, to better understand the terms used throughout this book.

Did you know? In parts of Asia, businessmen take long spa lunches to have their prostate milked during a massage. It is considered a good health practice in those cultures.

Terms, Types, and Stages of Orgasms

Massaging and adding pressure to the prostate brings a wide range of sensations and orgasms. Terminology varies from person, community, and culture. So consider that there is no universally agreed upon definition for orgasms.

Edging: The practice of engaging in sexual stimulation to the point of *almost* ejaculating, then stopping and starting again. This denial involves several repeated cycles of stimulation and is believed to lead to a more intense orgasm in the end.

Anal/Prostate Play: Covers stretching, depth training, prostate playing, etc. For the sake of simplicity, this term will be used to describe anal play sessions seeking anal/prostate orgasms.

Anal Orgasms/Prostate Orgasms: These terms will be used interchangeably. Anal orgasms can happen from simply touching the anus, stretching it, rimming, or deep penetration (anal nerve and muscle stimulation). Prostate orgasms occur when pressure or other types of stimulation are applied to the prostate. For simplicity, all the pleasure techniques in this book can be used for both anal and prostate orgasms.

Prostate Milking: Ejaculation but no orgasm. This is the one that is most commonly referred to in orgasm denial or chastity discussions. Usually, a finger or toy is inserted, and the prostate is massaged. This causes cum to flow out, caused by pressure on the prostate. There are no muscle contractions, no orgasms, and sometimes no pleasure. You effectively "urinate" the cum out. Some use the phrase "prostate milking" instead of prostate massage. Milking is forcing semen from the glands rather than them being emptied via orgasm and ejaculation. If you massage both seminal vesicles, prostate, and ampulla correctly, you could extract around 90 percent of the semen. Again, prostate milking has no climax pleasure, and you will have no semen release, only prostatic fluid. There will not be any penile contraction, you might not have an erection, and there is no refractory period. However, even without the pleasure of an orgasm, milking feels nice if you can do it.

Peegasm: Will sometimes occur when you have an anal orgasm and is caused by nerve stimulation in the bladder and pelvic region. A peegasm triggers your bladder and prostate simultaneously, sending lots of fluid through your penis. Usually, it is a mix of urine and prostatic fluid, with some semen. Nothing to fear. Just let your body's response happen and surrender to this pleasure if urine reflux occurs. This can be enjoyable and lead to seminal orgasms afterward, but it is best to spend time emptying your bladder before a session if you want to avoid these. But they are fun, albeit messy, and you can have several peegasms in a row; and they feel almost ejaculatory. Not to be confused with P-Gasms (prostate orgasms)—though peegasms often occur during a P-Gasm.

"Regular" Orgasm: A good old-fashioned penile orgasm caused by stimulating the penis until ejaculation occurs.

P-Waves: These involuntary contractions occur as pleasure waves that radiate from the area just below where you feel your bladder, right where your prostate gland is located. The feeling can be more subtle and dull, with euphoria that blooms and fades around the genital region. The electric sensations can be localized, spreading to other areas of your body near your prostate and penis, or further away from the source. They can be short or mid-length waves. The most intense P-Waves can be so powerful that they feel orgasmic and your prostate might throb or quiver, leading you to a dry orgasm, or Super-O (e.g., dry or wet prostate orgasms).

P-Gasms (prostate orgasms): An orgasm achieved through prostate stimulation, whether through direct contact (e.g., via penetration) or indirect means (e.g., kegel exercises, mental arousal, or external perineum pressure). P-Gasms occur when the prostate is the primary source of orgasmic sensation.

Dry (hands-free) Orgasm: Orgasm from P-Waves but without ejaculation. Also known as "hands-free dry orgasm"

(HFDO). These dry orgasms come from prostate stimulation, muscle contractions, mental focus, breathwork, or a combination. HFDOs can cause full-body contractions with incredible waves of pleasure that pulse throughout the body. These can be as intense as ejaculatory orgasms. Expect multiple waves of pleasure to rise and fall during this orgasm. There is no refractory period, meaning you can have several back-to-back HFDOs. Many seasoned veterans can have dry orgasms every 30 seconds nonstop for an hour or more. And they can begin within a few minutes of anal play. Dry orgasms can start mild, building to more intense ones that can lead to a Super-O.

Wet (hands-free) Orgasm: By definition, this means you ejaculate without rubbing or stimulating the penis. A "hands-free wet orgasm" (HFWO) results from stimulation of regions other than the penis. A HFWO can be considered a type of P-Gasm if the prostate is the primary source of orgasmic sensation. Some people can even have them with no prostate stimulation. Many use muscle contractions and fantasy or visualization to make this happen. For most, these orgasms are usually the result of anal stimulation. The wet orgasm happens when you massage the prostate with deep, hard strokes, and involuntarily force the cum out of it, causing an orgasm. Hands-free wet orgasms are more intense than traditional penile and anal dry orgasms. With practice, you can cum hands-free during prostate play, and some can have multiple wet orgasms, though this is rare. Firm pressure on the anterior (front) rectum or prostate will most likely lead to this. Some prefer to end the anal session at the peak of it with a rewarding, wet orgasm (through penile masturbation). Some prefer not to have a wet orgasm and let the sexual energy build for days.

Super Orgasm (Super-O): The ultimate orgasmic sensation. It provides energetic contractions all over the body at the same time. It brings altered states of consciousness with deep release. Some say it rejuvenates and brings profound spiritual experiences, not normally felt in regular penile orgasms. Some can last for as long as 15 minutes, where they keep getting stronger, pleasure after pleasure, and the waves continue growing. It usually starts with P-Gasms, waves of good warm tingly feelings up and around your body, then intensifies with longer waves, usually preceded by a series of dry orgasms. A Super-O is so intense that you feel the pleasure spread out to other parts of your body; it feels like your whole body is cumming. **It makes you feel like you are on drugs!** When you become more advanced, you will likely experience this continuous orgasm for long periods. It has a lot in common with female orgasms, causing full-body spasms and moaning for long periods. Along with HFWO, these are the holy grail of prostate play, sometimes accompanied by a wet orgasm, squirting, and other wet delights. A Super-O can be considered a type of P-Gasm if the prostate is the primary source of orgasmic sensation.

Super-T: This penile orgasm arrives after a HFDO (or several HFDOs) through penile masturbation; however, these are not the same as a traditional penile orgasm (typically without anal play). A Super-T is a concentrated, ejaculatory orgasm. As you are cumming, there are also several intervals of P-Waves that follow, sometimes creating more HFDOs. Highly recommended as a way to finish any anal session if you do not achieve a Super-O and need to release the built-up energy from powerful prostate sessions.

Blended Orgasm: Occurs both on a prostatic and ejaculatory level. Sometimes this happens during a Super-O session when the body orgasm awakes the nerve pathways that are connected to the pelvic region, causing the genitals to become uncontrollably stimulated and the penis to ejaculate.

Energy Orgasm (heart, nipple, vocal, full-body orgasms): These types of orgasms occur without touching any areas and are full-body. You use your breath and muscle contractions to generate orgasmic energy, flowing through the body. This too can result in Super-Os and ejaculation. Energy orgasms are the final chapter and the highest level in the anal pleasure category. They occur with mental practice and are considered a form of ecstatic mediation, the PhD or black belt level of anal play.

Erogenous Zone Orgasm: Some of you may cum with stimulation of the erogenous zones, such as nipples, ears, elbows, knees, neck, breasts, wrist, etc. These highly sensitive areas have more nerve endings, inducing different forms of orgasm. In conjunction with anal play, stimulating these areas can be a highly effective way to induce prostate orgasms. The right stimulation, however, varies from area to area and experience to experience—there is no single map for erogenous zones.

Tantra: A spiritual, philosophical tradition that integrates mindfulness, energy work, and sensuality to deepen connection with oneself and others. It emphasizes balance, consciousness, and the union of body, mind, and spirit. Neotantra is a modern, Western adaptation, focusing primarily on sensuality, intimacy, and personal growth rather than its original ritualistic aspects. It emphasizes mindfulness, energy flow, and conscious connection in relationships and sensuality.

Taoism: In terms of sexuality, this ancient philosophy focuses on cultivating vitality, longevity, and enlightenment. Taoist practices promote harmonizing masculine (Yang) and feminine (Yin) energies to enhance physical, emotional, and spiritual well-being. Techniques like controlled ejaculation, synchronized breathing, and energy circulation are designed to preserve sexual energy, rather than release it. The orgasm isn't just a momentary pleasure but a tool for deeper growth, intimacy, and cosmic unity.

K-Spot: Known as the kundalini spot, located behind the prostate. It is often described as a deeper extension of the perineal sponge. Stimulating this area can awaken kundalini energy, enhancing both pleasure and spiritual experiences. Tantric teachings suggest you can channel kundalini energy upward through the body (like a coiled snake), leading to more profound, transcendent orgasms.

Prostrainer/Prostranal: A prostrainer (noun) is an athlete constantly training and practicing for anal/prostate orgasms. Prostranal (verb or adjective) is the act of seeking and achieving anal/prostate orgasms.

Anal Physics: An equation I created that models the total mechanical energy contributing to arousal and orgasmic response based on variables of pleasure:

$$O = k \cdot \left(\int (S \cdot P \cdot F \cdot L)dt \right) + f(A, Ms, H, Bf)$$

Where:

- O = Orgasm likelihood/intensity

- k = Sensitivity coefficient (individual-dependent)

- S = Speed of thrust

- P = Pressure applied

- F = Frequency of thrust

- L = Depth of penetration

- A, Ms, H, Bf are arousal, mental state, hormones, and blood flow

Don't over analyze it—this formula is all about fun! Just play around with the variables in your sessions, experiment, and discover your own path to pleasure.

Let's review the most important terms to remember. You will see these often, so they are worth a quick refresher:

P-Waves – Light pleasure waves that build up gradually. You can ride P-Waves for a long time, enjoying the build-up before reaching a full orgasm.

P-Gasm – Happens when the prostate is the primary source of orgasmic sensation. This orgasm comes from prostate stimulation, either directly (internally) or indirectly (perineum pressure, muscle contractions, mental arousal, etc.).

Dry (hands-free) Orgasm – A type of P-Gasm that is an intense prostate/anal orgasm without penis stimulation or ejaculation, also known as HFDO (hands-free dry orgasm). It can come from prostate stimulation and muscle contractions, but also from mental focus, energy work, breathwork, or a combination of these.

Wet (hands-free) Orgasm – A type of P-Gasm, a hands-free wet orgasm (HFWO) occurs when ejaculation happens from a prostate or anal orgasm without any penile stimulation.

Super Orgasm (Super-O) – A long, rolling prostate/anal orgasm that keeps going. It comes in waves and lasts much longer, often resulting in a series of stacked P-Gasms.>

CHAPTER 3

PHASES OF LEARNING

Overview
- The four phases of learning: awareness, exploration, mastery, and expansion.
- The staircase concept explains how we progress in pleasure—first by copying techniques, then by creating our own.
- Dear lazy motherfuckers . . . there's no helicopter or elevator ride to the top of prostate heaven. You gotta climb one step at a time.

Now that you know the basics, let's loosely outline the path ahead, and what you can look forward to encountering . . .

Phase I: Pelvic floor contractions lead to involuntary contractions. Expect to start having your first P-Waves and a few P-Gasms and HFDOs. This first stage is simply exploring your body and mind to find the "electric switch" that is connected to your prostate. Channeling this energy and converting it to pleasure might be a challenging phase in the beginning. **This requires rewiring your brain** to build new pathways for pleasure, activating the neural circuitry in your brain. In short, you teach your mind and body that you don't just need your penis for orgasmic pleasure. You turn the mind into the master, and your body into the slave. It takes time to turn your rectum into a pleasure palace, as well as finding your prostate, and the pleasure spots around it.

Phase II: Will be filled with more frequent and intense P-Gasms and HFDOs. You'll have P-Waves rise quicker, and you are able to have dry orgasms in less than 15-60 seconds. As you learn to string these together, **P-Gasms and HFDOs become more and more intoxicating. They last longer, and it feels like you are reaching the point of getting closer to wet orgasms.** You will have steady beads of precum during these sessions, and you will feel pleasure expand past your genital area, out to other parts of your body. Your mind becomes stronger, controlling more of the process. The body serves by being a conduit for increased pleasure. You'll likely even have long edging sessions with toys inside of you. This stage requires that you practice "ruined orgasms".

Ruined orgasms are precisely as their name suggests. The process involves moving toward a peak of pleasure, only to deliberately interrupt it before it fully develops. This shares certain characteristics with the practice of edging, where the orgasm is stopped right before full climax. This act is repeated several times before finally permitting a full release. You will learn how to have Super-T orgasms, and your regular penile orgasms become stronger and longer as well. Your interest in doing the sexual things you once enjoyed might diminish. You might also start having prostate sessions before you have sex with your partner; and you will want a toy inside of you during sex.

Phase III: Expect light showers and the possibility of torrential wetness. With the steady practice of kegels (anal contractions), you will finally get to the wet stage and go from a prostrainer to a "prosdrainer". This is when it gets mind-blowing . . . you finally get to experience what some women can do: squirt! There are 3 types of liquid emissions you might experience. The first and easiest one to produce is prostatic fluid. This is a form of prostate milking and often leaks out with semen, but it is orgasmic. It looks clear to milky and is often sweet and slightly salty and even might have a musky smell. The other liquid you will squirt is a mix of urine and/or semen. It looks like pee but might also have a mix of semen and prostatic fluid; this is typically considered a peegasm.

Lastly, **expect to have semen erupt** if you are fortunate enough to have a HFWO. You should also be experiencing Super-Os during this phase. Remember: during this "wetter" phase, do not be scared to release. It feels like you need to pee. Do not hold back. Let the fluids out and enjoy the pleasure that comes from their release. This skill helps you fine tune how to activate a HFWO.

As you progress and master your practice, you could be having wet orgasms in less than 10 minutes. This is the phase I am in now. My sessions can range anywhere from 15 minutes to 1 hour. I usually have a few prostatic releases, then finish with 1 or 2 wet orgasms. Even though I cum, I still feel aroused afterward, and need to have a wet penile orgasm later. Despite the physical release of semen, this stage leaves you with more erections throughout the day and a sense of needing more anal stimulation. It drives your sexual energy even higher. So be warned! Each contraction and orgasm build a hunger, craving, and desire that even a penile orgasm can't relieve. In this phase, you will master the Super-T and find it helpful when you are unable to achieve Super-Os.

You will probably be in your bedroom alone for hours every day exploring all the possibilities of your prostate. Your partner might become more involved by incorporating it into your sex life. You could become addicted to prostate play for a while. It also raises the level of lovemaking with your partner.

Phase IV: A new chapter begins. Expect darkness to turn to light in this Jedi phase. The prostrainer student has learned so much, including that there is so much more to learn. The easy stages of anal pleasure have been conquered, but the limitless journey has just begun. This last phase of anal orgasms focuses on blended and/or energy orgasms. These spiritual levels are the highest form of anal orgasms. They can bring both dry and wet orgasms simply from mental practice and ecstatic meditation. Some describe it as a never-ending Super-O, lasting for hours. We are talking transcendental-level shit here! **You might cum so hard that your molecules get transported to another dimension in time and space.** And some prostainers can do this without kegels (anal contractions) or anal stimulation—only using their mind. This is the 10th-degree black belt of Tantra. Penile orgasms feel the same as Super-Os. And you are able to repeat each of them on command, making the pleasure endlessly last as long as you want. You might even become complacent doing it regularly. If so, save yourself for special sessions, letting your sexual energy build for weeks. You and your partner now have more tantric sex, and slower prostate sessions.

Note: These stages are the "typical" progression and will vary for everyone. Do not expect them necessarily to be linear.

For many, the first anal orgasm will be a dry one. It will start with learning to feel P-Waves radiating from your prostate. At first, the P-Waves will rise faintly during anal play, then fade away and become a distant echo. Over time, they will become more pronounced and last longer. Once you master this stage, you will begin to form precum and have dry orgasms that will feel like phantom wet orgasms. These will leave you twitching and gasping for air. And you might even look down thinking you came!

The Staircase

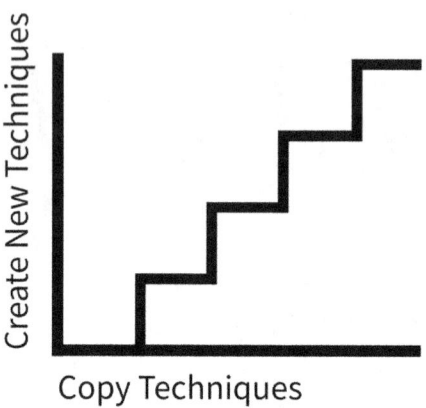

The staircase concept provides a simple framework for understanding how we approach pleasure and evolve toward prostate orgasms. Think of the horizontal line below the staircase as a direction where you "copy" techniques. This could be from copying a prostate technique in my book, something you read or watched online. Little by little, you make progress and move forward, but not up. This horizontal progress focuses on gradual improvements and refinements to enhance your existing experiences of pleasure. This is essentially a case of "monkey see, monkey do". These incremental changes can lead to a more reliable increase in pleasure, but you stay within the bounds of what you already know. This is simply following directions.

The vertical line, however, is where the steps of rapid learning and growth take place. It represents upward progress, which involves big shifts that redefine your relationship with pleasure and take your experiences to entirely new heights on the staircase. This could be creating new positions/angles, experimenting with timing, or introducing new fantasies. You are not copying here. You are an innovator of anal play. A learning mindset turns into a mastermind. You start looking for technical breakthroughs that transform how you experience and perceive pleasure. It unlocks levels of satisfaction and intimacy that are revolutionary to your skill set. **Good prostrainers copy. But great prostrainers innovate.**

The journey to reliable prostate orgasms combines both copying techniques and creating new ones. Building the foundation involves mastering the basics of your arousal and response cycle, experimenting with gradual enhancements, and discovering what works best for you—and what doesn't. Creating new techniques means breaking free from routine and aiming for radical experiences by looking at old situations with a fresh perspective.

The ultimate goal is to go as high as you can on the staircase, breaking every ceiling along the way. You want to move beyond routine pleasure toward groundbreaking orgasms, seeking profound experiences that engage your mind, body, and spirit. This isn't just about "achieving a prostate orgasm"—it's about embracing a lifestyle where pleasure becomes a boundless force of self-discovery.

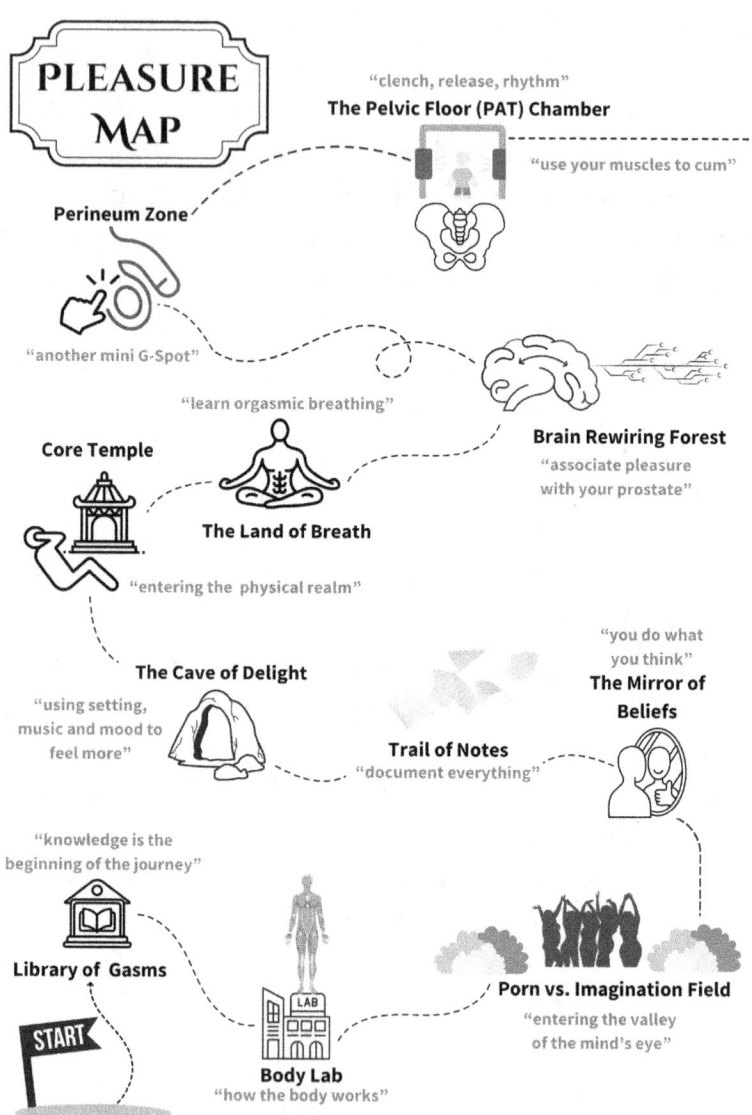

PLEASURE MAP

"clench, release, rhythm"
The Pelvic Floor (PAT) Chamber

"use your muscles to cum"

Perineum Zone

"another mini G-Spot"

"learn orgasmic breathing"

Brain Rewiring Forest
"associate pleasure with your prostate"

Core Temple

The Land of Breath

"entering the physical realm"

The Cave of Delight

"you do what you think"
The Mirror of Beliefs

"using setting, music and mood to feel more"

Trail of Notes
"document everything"

"knowledge is the beginning of the journey"

Library of Gasms

START

Porn vs. Imagination Field
"entering the valley of the mind's eye"

LAB

Body Lab
"how the body works"

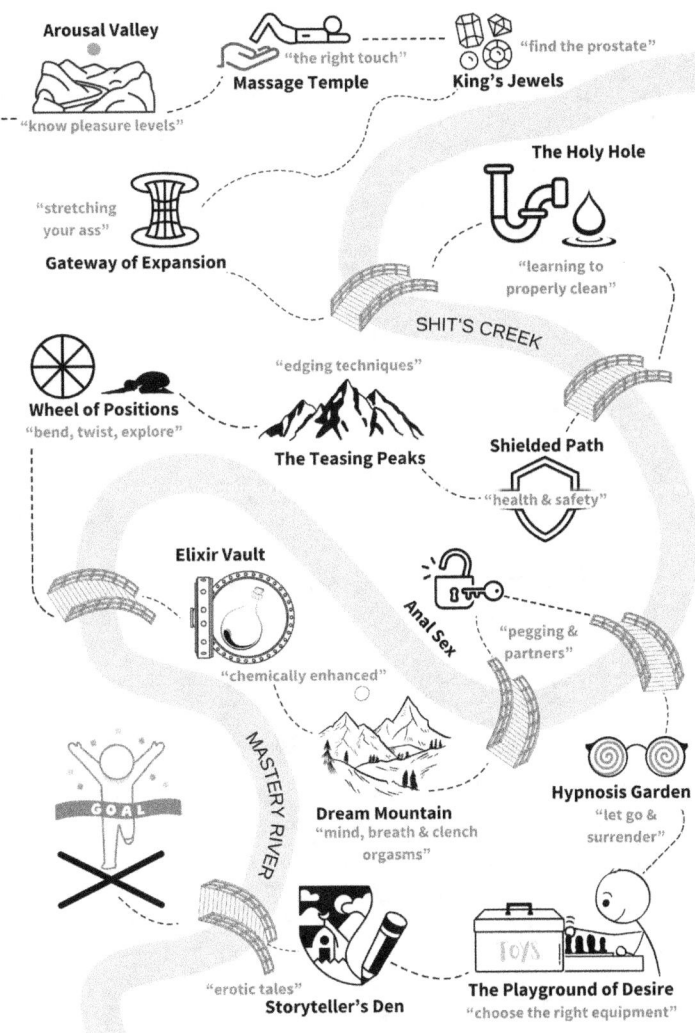

Here's a sneak peek of what's ahead. Your learning journey is a lot like following a wild, winding treasure map! You can bounce around like a pirate chasing shiny loot, but if you want to become a true master, I'd suggest sticking to the trail.

CHAPTER 4

ANATOMY AND SCIENCE OF ANAL PLEASURE

Overview
- Learn how nerves and muscles work together to create pleasure.
- Discover how stimulation activates the body's natural orgasm response.
- Relax—you're not in med school, and there's no test. Just enjoy the scenery.

Located inside the rectum, the prostate rests between the penis and bladder, while the urethra runs through the center of it. **The prostate is a walnut-sized gland roughly 1-3 inches inside the anus,** located between the bladder and rectum. Locate your prostate upwards and toward the front of your groin. With your finger inserted, you find it by scooping inward, slightly toward your perineal area. You will feel a firm, raised surface.

The prostate supports the reproductive system by providing a fluid coating for semen (ejaculate). The prostate muscles act like a "cum sump pump" to help push semen through your urethra. The prostate is mainly made up of two types of tissues: one that acts like a gland, and another that's more like muscles and connective fibers. This gland part is surrounded by a thin layer, which is kind of like a coating; the tissue wraps around big blood vessels. This is one of the reasons it can be so sensitive. Thousands of nerve endings surround the prostate area. After stimulation of these prostatic nerves, an activation of the sympathetic nerves occurs resulting in a powerful orgasm. This can be accompanied by an emission of semen, prostatic fluid, and/or urine.

> Did you know? Skene's glands are the equivalent of the female prostate. They reside along the female urethra. These glands secrete fluid that helps with urination and provide fluid for female ejaculation and/or lubrication during sex.

The prostate gets signals from nerves in the body that help with different functions such as pleasure and ejaculation. **When you orgasm from your penis, certain nerves activate the muscles in the prostate.** These important bundles of nerves and blood vessels near the prostate help with erections. They're like wires and pipes that run through the penis.

The prostate is divided into three areas:

- **Central Zone**: This is the center area around the tubes that carry sperm.
- **Transitional Zone**: This part surrounds the tube you pee through. It can sometimes grow larger in a

non-cancerous way, causing urinary problems.

- **Peripheral Zone:** This is the biggest part. It is mostly at the back. The tubes here are more open to letting urine flow back, and that can cause inflammation. Prostate cancer is often found in this area. The peripheral zone is mainly the area felt against the rectum and known as the pleasure spot.

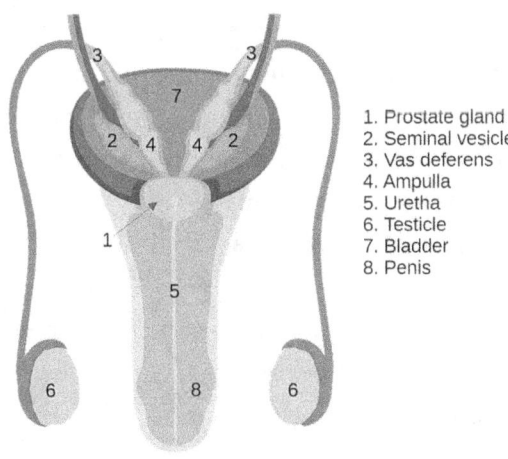

1. Prostate gland
2. Seminal vesicle
3. Vas deferens
4. Ampulla
5. Uretha
6. Testicle
7. Bladder
8. Penis

Front view of the reproductive/urogenital system.

Anal stimulation tricks the body into activating your cum sump pump, priming your prostate to fill with fluid, and experiencing the same feeling as ejaculating. This dry orgasm feeling is a very unique experience. It tricks the prostate into filling with as much (prostatic) fluid as possible. This fluid can build up in the prostate causing intense pressure to form. By arousing the prostate, it's possible to release the prostatic fluid without ejaculating and replicate the sensation of an orgasm. Applying pressure to your prostate can produce sensations similar to a traditional penile orgasm. This becomes an infinite loop of pleasure because dry prostate orgasms require a shorter refractory period (recovery time) than a regular penile wet orgasm. And you can have several of them! Learning to experience this can transform your relationship with your body.

Think about the prostate as a sponge trying to fill with water. You squeeze the sponge a little bit so that it can soak up more water. **You trick the prostate into making more fluid so that the feeling of cumming, or needing to cum, keeps going for as long as you can handle it.** Since dry orgasms make the prostate fill with fluid, it is not uncommon for the prostatic fluid and semen to leak (milking).

After a penile orgasm (ejaculation), the semen reservoir will fully refill in 2-3 days, possibly sooner for a healthy, younger person with high libido. Any edging and/or teasing builds up sexual tension, thus creating more semen. The whole point of waiting to cum is to have your semen reservoir full so you can achieve prostate orgasms easier and feel them stronger.

The same goes for prostatic fluid. **If you experiment with anal play often, you will have less prostatic fluid, and the nerves in your anal area becomes more desensitized.** This requires that you figure out the right schedule for your body, so you can play regularly while also maintaining sensitivity for Super-Os.

The organs in your lower pelvis, such as your bladder and colon, are supported by a large group of muscles called the pelvic floor muscles. Working with your anal sphincter, the pelvic floor muscles help you stop embarrassing gas and stool leaks. These internal muscles (your sphincter, the pubococcygeus (PC) muscle, and the pelvic floor muscles) help induce an anal orgasm. **By rapidly tensing and relaxing, you can bring a full-body sensation that radiates throughout the body, making it feel like your entire body is climaxing.**

Your internal sphincter is an involuntary muscle. This means you cannot consciously control it. Similar to your beating heart or your diaphragm, the sphincter does its job every second of the day without realizing its always at work. The internal sphincter is programmed to stay shut. You can, however, control your external sphincter muscles with practice. This is done by learning to control your pelvic floor muscles, which will be discussed in detail in an upcoming chapter. The key to having anal orgasms is learning to freely control these areas.

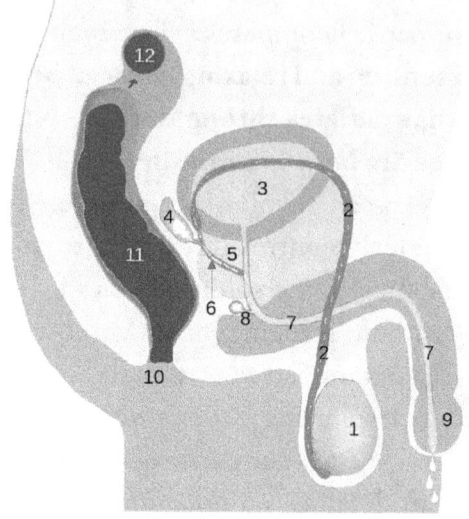

1. Testicles
2. Vas deferens
3. Bladder (urine)
4. Seminal vesicle
5. Prostate gland
6. Ejaculatory duct
7. Uretha
8. Cowper's gland
9. Penis
10. Anus
11. Rectum
12. Colon sigmoideum

Side view of the reproductive/urogenital system showing the "cum highway". Testicles are where the sperm is made. During ejaculation, it travels in the vas deferens duct, through the prostate. The seminal vesicles and prostate gland add fluids to nourish and support the sperm, forming semen. The semen then passes through the ejaculatory duct into the urethra, which runs through the penis, and is expelled during ejaculation.

The chamber inside the prostate is connected to the seminal vesicles (aka the main source of semen). And the vas deferens is the highway that transports sperm from the testicles. The ampulla of vas deferens, also known as the ampulla of ductus deferens, is a widened section of the vas deferens located at the base of the bladder; this acts as a holding tank for sperm. Semen is made of the fluid that is produced by the prostate. Sperm is produced in the testes. Muscle contractions during sex push out both. Some of the fluid pushes from vesicles before the orgasm, and contains almost none to little sperm, aka precum.

When stimulated directly, the prostate can generate cum without ejaculation; even without an erection being present. For most, this takes time, effort, and expertise to happen. Because the prostate can be pleasurably manipulated inside the rectum, prostate-related orgasms can occur regularly and be repeated.

> Imagine cumming over and over in pure bliss for an hour from anal orgasms!

To put it bluntly, you are placing pressure on the prostate and seminal vesicles. This creates stimulation and gets the juices flowing. In fact, your clear prostatic fluid is similar to female squirt fluid. This seminal fluid can easily be produced and several squirtings can occur once you find the right spots. The pubococcygeus muscle and prostatic milking can be achieved by learning to apply and squeeze with intense pressure. When you hit the prostate gland, it triggers the urinary, ejaculate, and causes an incredible feeling. Depending on the type of orgasm you experience, it feels like you are peeing and ejaculating at the same time. For many, the initial feeling of a peeing sensation is a good sign—it means you found the right spot.

And there are even more vast riches in this area! An anal orgasm intensely stimulates the sigmoid colon (or sigmorectal junction), triggering a pushing action that leads to release and contractions. The anal region is packed with nerves, making exploration an incredibly pleasurable experience. You can still achieve orgasm by stimulating these nerves, even without directly targeting the prostate. Sensations from this region are primarily carried by the pudendal and sacral nerves—plus, don't forget to thank your vagus nerve, which is also nearby. Hitting these pathways can create intense euphoria and even lightheaded states.

Learning to do pelvic floor muscle exercises (also called kegels) will help stimulate the prostate, pudendal, and perineal nerves and associated muscles. The pudendal and perineal nerves run just outside of the scrotum from the head of the penis to the inguinal canal (groin tunnel). The nerves are a bundled string between the testicles and legs. The pudendal nerve is the main nerve of the perineum. It carries sensation from the outside genitalia of both sexes, and the skin around the anus and perineum, as well as the motor supply to various pelvic muscles. This includes the external sphincter areas in both biological sexes.

In fact, the whole digestive tract, from your mouth to the anus, is lined with its own nervous system. This is known as the enteric nervous system (ENS), which is more complex than even the spinal cord. The INS (aka, intrinsic nervous system) is one of the main divisions of the entire nervous system. It consists of a mesh-like system of neurons that controls the function of the gastrointestinal tract. It is capable of acting independently of the sympathetic and parasympathetic nervous systems. And did you know that your gut produces 95% of the body's serotonin? Serotonin is your body's vibe manager—boosting mood, pleasure, and gut flow to keep you feeling good.

We tend to accumulate lots of stress and anxiety in this area. Emotions and memories can be stored in the tissues.

Since the ENS is interconnected, **your first anal orgasm could unlock deep emotions and trauma.**

CHAPTER 5

THE MECHANICS OF ANAL ORGASMS

Overview

- Create the right mindset and environment to enhance pleasure and deepen sensations.
- Relaxation, breathing, and a strong core improve orgasm potential.
- Track progress with a journal to refine techniques and recognize patterns.
- Explore sound arousal, nipple play, perineum play, and semen retention for deeper pleasure.
- Rewiring the body and mind takes commitment and belief.
- This chapter is all about setting the stage for success.

The phrase "neurons that fire together, rewire together" means that when certain brain cells (neurons) work together, often they'll form stronger connections. This helps us create habits, feelings, and behaviors. For example, if you regularly exercise and feel happy afterward, your brain starts to link the two things.

Over time, the more you exercise, the more natural it becomes to feel happy afterward, and the stronger this habit becomes.

Our brain is made up of different parts that do different jobs, but they work together. When parts of the brain that control actions and emotions fire at the same time, they create new habits and feelings. For instance, if you practice breathing deeply when you feel stressed, your brain connects deep breathing with feeling calm. This helps you stay at peace more easily in the future. By repeating these actions, you can change your habits and experiences, helping you feel and act in new and beneficial ways.

Orgasms are complex experiences that involve an alignment of the right nerve stimulation, proper rhythmic stimulation, syncing of breath, and emotional connection (open mind and open heart).

Cumming from anal takes time, practice, experimentation, and the right tools. It took me several toys and patience to reach strong, dry orgasms. Everyone's timeline will be different. Your body and sexual responses operate independently, so do not compare it with other prostrainers.

The first step is creating the perfect environment for positive feedback loops, allowing you to ride the waves of sensation and fully surrender to the experience. **Eventually, you will realize that the mind can either rob your pleasure or help you achieve new levels of pleasure.** Arousal isn't just about physical stimulation; it's about how the mind perceives, anticipates, and amplifies pleasure. By learning to harness these feedback loops—through breath control, muscle engagement, and mental focus—you can turn arousal into an ever-expanding cycle, unlocking deeper and more immersive pleasure experiences.

Making small incremental improvements every day can lead to great breakthroughs. No one learns to have an anal orgasm overnight. It happens with trial and error, regular practice, and determination.

Ultimately, this process requires you to learn to control the mind. Imagine it as a ladder. If intrusive thoughts take over, you go down a few steps. If you start the session with too much stress, you probably won't even find the ladder. With prostate play, you must master breathing, relaxation, and mental clarity.

As you read this book, remember that **everyone brings their own unique experiences and backgrounds**. Some of you may have already spent years exploring different approaches to anal play, while others may be new to this journey. Regardless of where you are, this book offers multiple opportunities for exploration and presents several variations on technique and philosophy.

The following sections focus on fundamental skills that you can experiment with as you feel more comfortable going deeper into your practice. You will encounter more advanced techniques and concepts that build upon these basic skills later in the book. It's worth noting that all of the material presented is based on personal experience, research, and discussions with others.

Technique Playbook

> Relax and focus on the sensations, not the orgasm!

As you are reading this right now, take a second to check in with yourself and notice how your body feels. Are your shoulders tense, your breath shallow, or your mind racing with thoughts? Or perhaps you feel calm, grounded, and at ease. This awareness is the first step in understanding the powerful role your nervous system plays into prostate play. The autonomic nervous system constantly regulates your body's responses to stress and relaxation. Understanding how these systems work can empower you to take control of your well-being and restore balance, even in the midst of chaotic life.

The calming of the nervous system leads to relaxation. The parasympathetic nervous system (PNS) turns on when the body is slowed down and at rest. Conversely, the sympathetic nervous system (SNS) controls your body's responses to perceived threats and is responsible for "fight or flight" responses. Being aware of what state you're in is important, but it is even more critical to know how to switch your body to a parasympathetic state.

The following practices will shift you into a parasympathetic state and get you ready for prostate play:

- **Do not rush** – Slow down. Prostate play can take a long time, especially at first. Set aside a good amount of time to explore the sensation and identify what feels pleasurable. Do not attempt it knowing you have to meet someone in an hour, or you know your roommate will be home soon, and so on.

- **Get in the mood** – Adjust your setting with lighting, music, and other things that can elevate the mood. I recommend starting with some online guided meditations, especially if you had a very stressful day, or regularly experience anxiety. Use this time to tune into your body holistically. Dressing up is a personal choice. Many prefer being naked. But some like to wear a sexy outfit, or even lingerie, for their anal sessions.
- **Stimulate multiple areas** – Try some foreplay. Start by touching erogenous zones, including the genitals. Focusing on multiple body parts helps you reach orgasm and makes the experience even more powerful. There are so many ways to trigger pleasure from touching sensitive skin areas, massaging your muscles, playing with the nipples, and the genitalia area. Relax into the pleasure and gently touch your body wherever it feels good. Or use a feather.
- **Visualize** – Close your eyes and imagine sexual thoughts. Fantasize about having an anal orgasm. Scientific evidence highlights the role of imagining sexual stimulation, and how this can increase the likelihood of reaching an orgasm. Listening to hypnotic audio files, and following the voice with your eyes closed, elevates your experience and sends you into a trance state (explore shibbydex.com). You can also watch videos of others having hands-free anal orgasms or read erotic stories.
- **Sound** – Use earbuds/headphones or play music to

block out unwanted sounds. There are many options for enhancing your sessions. (*See the following section for more details.*)

The trickiest part of prostate play is staying focused on what you want to accomplish. It's easy for your mind to wander, especially while building your orgasm. The solution? Stay focused, fully immerse yourself in the moment. Begin by anchoring your attention to the sensations in your body—notice the rhythm of your breath, the heat of your skin, and the way energy flows and builds. Focus on a fantasy as vividly as possible. If your mind starts to wander, gently guide it back to these sensations without judgment, and slow your breath down to help ground you.

Pinpoint exactly where it feels good. Visualize the pleasure as a wave you're riding, allowing it to crest naturally without rushing or holding back. You can also use a mantra like, "I welcome this building sensation." or "I love the feeling of pleasure." Remember, the key is to let go of distractions and surrender to the intensity of the present moment, trusting your body to lead the way.

Porn vs. Imagination

Some have trouble getting turned on and need porn to get aroused. Others prefer to create fantasies in their own mind. Or it can be a mixture of both. Either way, getting into a sexual trance state is deeply personal. Determine what works best to get you aroused, then incorporate this into your play sessions.

If you do have a tendency to prefer porn, take a second to think about what your brain is doing in that mode: is it constantly seeking "weak" dopamine hits every second and scene? The answer is probably yes. Typically, porn floods your brain with an unlimited supply of its own addictive chemicals. The instant gratification loop it gives keeps us from experiencing higher levels of orgasmic pleasure. This doesn't mean you have to give up porn—just make an effort to cut back.

Achieving a heightened full-body prostate orgasm requires focus and attempting to multitask—trying to juggle multiple sensations or thoughts at once—can be a major obstacle. For beginners, dividing your attention between too many stimuli can weaken the intensity of the experience and make it harder to reach that peak state. Mastery begins with tuning out distractions. You are directing your mental and physical energy into focused awareness, allowing you to discover the subtle sensations within your body.

Remember, porn can never outshine the creativity of your own imagination. Your brain has the ability to stream content that exceeds anything a studio can produce. Don't get me wrong, porn can be fantastic when you need a little jumpstart to get aroused at the beginning of a session. But when you are starting out on your prostate journey, it's best to take breaks from it occasionally.

Pleasing yourself without porn forces you to think and ask yourself, "What exactly turns me on right now?" This is the essence of true sexual freedom. In prostate play, you are trying to figure out what works and what doesn't work. Having a play session without porn allows creativity to happen. It lets you to craft your own fantasies and scenes based on your individual sexual tastes. It helps you climb the staircase to new levels; and you **create the "strong" dopamine hits by using your imagination and focusing on where your pleasure points**

are located. Tapping into the power of your expansive mind, and leveraging the chemicals in your brain, will unlock deeper emotional and physical sensations.

There is certainly no single "right" way to play. It's important to unlock your desires, approaching prostate play in a way that feels enjoyable and safe for you. I'm merely reminding you that you don't need to rely on porn for positive stimulus. You're an incredible human being with boundless imagination. It's a beautiful gift. Use it often and freely.

And if you do decide to default to porn, I recommend watching other prostrainers. There is nothing like seeing someone having a hands-free orgasm to get inspired! Or get a mirror and use your camera to record your session up close. Making your own porn could help you to move beyond the self-consciousness of prostate play, turning it into an empowering and hot experience. Just make sure you delete or encrypt it afterwards, especially if you have snooping family members or roommates in the household.

Manifesting It

Before beginning any session, take a moment to clearly define your intention. This isn't about pressuring yourself to achieve a specific result—it's about setting a course, like charting your boat to a distant island that you can see on the horizon. Whether your goal is to "experience a dry orgasm" or simply "feel relaxed and aroused", stating it consciously helps align your mind and body. It sends a clear signal to the universe about your desire. At the same time, let go of any attachment—don't expect anything to happen! This paradoxical state is crucial: it reduces anxiety while keeping the door open for greater things to happen.

Think of it as planting a seed of possibility. You're not forcing an outcome but creating a setting that allows your session to unfold naturally. And you create certainty in this uncertain space by how you react to the evolving session with your intention. For instance, when I was starting out, I'd set simple intentions for each individual session. I started by saying things to myself such as, "I am going to have a P-Gasm every 30 seconds for 20 minutes." This was achievable for me and helped build my confidence. In fact, many times I ended up overachieving my intention and discovered new breakthroughs.

Week after week, my intentions and goals evolved. Later on, I started by saying, "I easily squirt precum." Sure enough, a rope of precum/prostatic fluid shot out during my session, and it felt amazing. Fast forward, I remember the day I had my first full hands-free wet orgasm (Super-O). For two weeks, I came so close. I was repeating to myself over and over, "I easily have a HFWO." I would tell myself this while driving, while having prostate sessions, and when I was falling asleep at night. This repetitive statement grew stronger and louder in my head. I knew it was going to happen—and sure enough, it did. I kept repeating my intention in my mind, convincing myself that it was bound to happen. That alignment between my intention and action created the perfect conditions for success.

> "There is only consciousness and awareness. Whatever you are aware of being, you become." — Neville Goddard

Turn up the BAS

Remember these three elevated emotions: Belief, Acceptance, and Surrender. **Believe you can cum from anal. Accept and embrace your physical body. And surrender to the sensations when they arise.** This is how you change your internal state and get the results you desire. The opposite is succumbing to fear, doubt, anger, insecurity, judgment, anxiety, shame, etc. Do not let these emotions take hold during your practice and journey. Disappointment happens when we are pressuring ourselves with expectations. Then we flood ourselves with negative thinking. This is where you need to be a mental warrior. For every one good thought, there are usually 100 bad thoughts. So you need to fight through this and become aware of your thinking at all times.

Changing your beliefs and perceptions will bring you to a new state of pleasure. What unconscious thoughts have you been agreeing to? And which ones hold you back? If you repeat a mental attitude, you create a belief. The redundancy of your thoughts over time conditions your body. I'm asking you do something different here. **Let go of any old beliefs that are holding you back from embracing a new future of limitless pleasure**.

But remember, just changing your beliefs and perceptions a few times is not enough—you have to reinforce that change again and again, over and over, until your neurons fire in new ways, rewiring your physiology. You have to be a fierce soldier every day to defeat the old you. Like a pickleball player who practices their backhand over and over until they master it.

A focused intention must be a part of your plan of action. You must learn to order your mind, to create clarity from entropy, and to establish a routine practice. This is how you make progress and get into the flow state. This allows your body and mind to provide feedback, confirming that you're making progress toward your goals, so you climb up the stairway to prostate heaven faster.

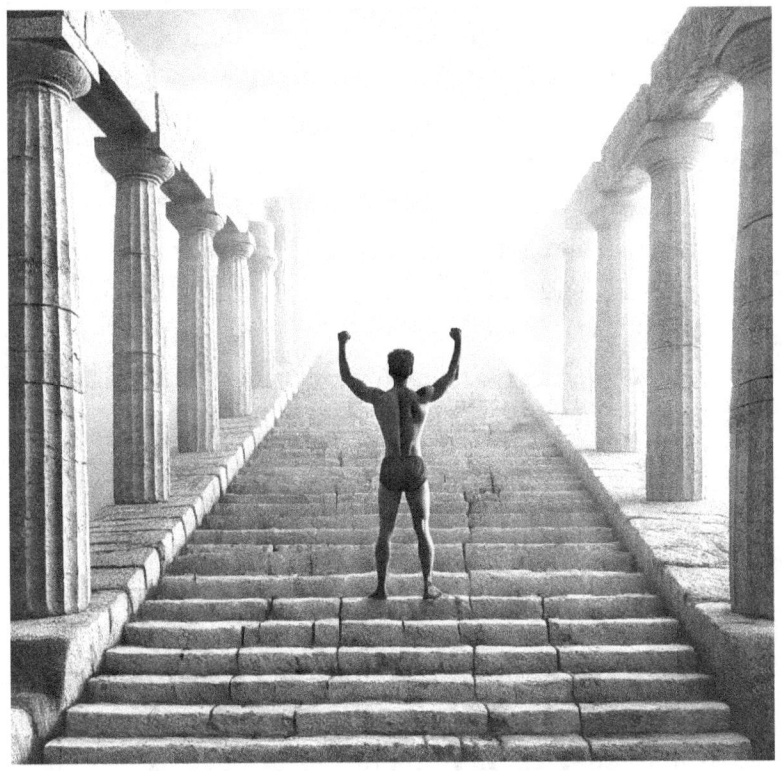

Create a mental positive feedback loop. Your intention creates clarity. Clarity speeds up the process. This speed will generate progress. Progress drives flow. And flow leads to infinite prostate orgasms.

Declaration of Intention

There came a point where I said to myself, "I have prostate orgasms!" every morning. Additionally, I visualized what it felt and looked like so that every single detail was fantasized. The music that was playing. The smell of the room. The emotions I was feeling, and so on. I even wrote it down on my yearly goals list in front of my bathroom mirror: "HFWO". I didn't use the future tense, "I will." Instead, I acted as if it had already happened. This is the level of dedication you need to have!

Grab a pen and get ready to write. It is time to create your own commitment and belief statement. Create a paragraph stating how you are going to accomplish your goal of learning how to have prostate orgasms. Write an aggressive declaration. For example:

I have prostate orgasms. I feel the pleasure of cumming hands-free. I practice daily, weekly, and as long as necessary. I achieve this state of bliss. My belief is so strong that nothing can stop me! I give up negative thinking, and laziness; primarily masturbating with my hand . . . I cum from anal!

Be fun and creative. Make your statement as long or as short as you want.

Do not get stuck into thinking "I can't!" This mentality leads you to quit without trying the exercises, because you've already told yourself it's not going to work. And do not get stuck into saying "I will", as it makes it less immediate and unlikely to happen. Like anything in life, success requires a shift in mindset and unwavering conviction. This keeps you progressing, even when faced with obstacles.

Read your newly written statement every day, and before

you have a prostate session. Visualize yourself having these prostate orgasms. Imagine the place, the time of day, what the room looks like, the toy you are using. Imagine the sensations and mentally feel the emotions. Tell yourself everyday, "I have prostate orgasms!" This is a big part of your success.

Becoming an Analyst

Embrace the role of a scientist and document your journey. Keeping an improvement journal allows you to approach your exploration with the precision of a field scientist. A journal becomes your personal lab notebook where you record your experiences, track progress, and note discoveries. Whether it's a structured log or a free-form diary, documenting your journey allows you to identify patterns, refine techniques, and gain insights into what works best for your body and mind. Just as scientists rely on data to draw conclusions, you can use your entries to guide and improve your practice. This is what gets you to the new levels on the staircase.

With a journal, you can track, analyze, and adapt along the way. Capture the variety of details—moods, sensations, techniques, intentions, and outcomes in a session. Create a treasure trove of data that reveals your unique patterns over time. For example, you might notice that certain techniques (e.g., depth of the toy, vibration patterns, etc.) consistently lead to deeper experiences, or you discover that setting specific intentions enhances your sessions. Logging details such as the time of day, mindset, or even your diet and sleep could provide surprising insights. By treating each entry as a valuable data point, you empower yourself to adapt your approach based on real evidence rather than guesswork *(see "Your Cyborg*

Ass: Tech and Sex Toys, Data-Driven Desire" section for a list of self-pleasure tracker apps).

Here are some potential columns and rows to add in your journal/tracker:

- **Date** – The date of the session for tracking patterns over time. (e.g., weekdays might be better).
- **Time of Day** – Morning, afternoon, or evening to identify optimal times.
- **Mood/Emotion** – How you felt before starting (e.g., relaxed, stressed, excited).
- **Intention** – What you aimed to achieve (e.g., relaxation, HFDO, connection).
- **Techniques Used** – Specific methods or practices during the session.
- **Duration** – Length of the session.
- **Environment** – Notes about the setting (e.g., location, lighting, temperature, scents).
- **Partnered or Solo** – Indicate if the session involved a partner or was solo.
- **Physical Sensations** – Key sensations experienced (e.g., tingling, warmth, intensity).
- **Equipment** – Types used (e.g., Aneros, e-stim, lube).
- **Emotional Response** – How you felt during or after (e.g., joy, frustration, connection).
- **Sensitivity** – Detail how it felt before, during, and after (e.g., sore, extra sensitive, numb).
- **Breakthroughs** – Any new experiences or achievements.
- **Challenges** – What didn't work or felt difficult.
- **Arousal Level (1–10)** – A self-assessed score

for arousal.

- **Outcome** – Results achieved (e.g., orgasm type, relaxation, energy shift).
- **Energy Levels Before/After** – Rate your energy levels pre- and post-session.
- **Experimentation Notes** – Observations about new approaches or variations.
- **Partner Feedback** – Insights or input from a partner, if applicable.
- **Reflections** – Free-form notes about insights or thoughts.
- **Next Steps** – Ideas for future sessions or areas to focus on.

Sometimes, structured tracking isn't enough to capture the details of your journey. A free-form journaling session can provide a deeper, more intuitive perspective. Write about how you felt before, during, and after a session; or explore emotions and thoughts that arise in the process. This unstructured reflection can uncover hidden blocks, untapped desires, or moments of unexpected clarity. Over time, reviewing these entries can help you see growth that might otherwise go unnoticed, and it keeps you connected to your goals. The combination of structured data and free journaling creates a holistic picture of your journey, blending the analytical and the emotional for better self-discovery.

Keep checking your progress and reread your entries—it helps you get better step by step. Like the old saying goes, "The road to mastery is built on measurement."

Sound Arousal

Not only does sound help with relaxation, it can also be a tool to help you reach high-levels of arousal. There is something uniquely satisfying about tapping into your own imagination with the help of sound arousal. **Erotic audio makes the canvas of your mind come alive**. Since so much of prostate play is tied to the mental stimulation, audio can really rev up your central nervous system and increase prostate orgasms.

Welcome to this guide on audio practices and stimulation techniques. As you dive into these arousal amplification methods, it's important to understand that you're not obligated to adopt every single one. Instead, think of this as a buffet of options where you're free to select what suits you best. Each technique is like a different flavor awaiting your exploration, and your task is to test and discover which resonates most with your preferences, needs, and circumstances. So go for it—explore, experiment, and find what feels best for you! Remember, it's all up to you. This book is your adventure—pick the techniques that make your journey worthwhile.

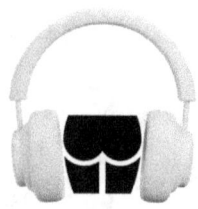

Mediation sounds: These calming audio files, like chants, nature sounds, or soft ambient music, help boost relaxation and potentially increase orgasmic experiences. They let you achieve deep states of calm. The key is to also try other exercises while listening, such as practicing mindfulness or deep breathing. This strongly triggers the body's relaxation response, lowering heart rate and reducing stress hormones. The right soundscape creates an ideal setting that promotes relaxation, allowing the mind and body to unwind, setting the stage for increased sensitivity to pleasurable sensations. This combined practice helps reduce anxiety, which can be a barrier to sexual arousal.

By calming the mind and promoting a sense of calm, meditation sounds create an environment that encourages heightened sensory perception. This heightened awareness of bodily sensations, combined with a serene auditory backdrop, fosters a greater mind-body connection, potentially contributing to more orgasmic responses.

There are many types of meditation sounds that you can explore on **Spotify** or **YouTube**. Some of my favorites include sound bowl healing, ocean sounds, and Tibetan chanting. Individual experiences, based on personal preferences, may vary with these techniques.

Binaural beats / specific frequencies: Often measured in hertz (Hz) or megahertz (MHz), they have been suggested to impact brainwave patterns and potentially influence mental states. Binaural beats are created by presenting two slightly different frequencies to each ear. The brain perceives a third tone, the binaural beat, which is the difference between the two presented frequencies. Different (specific) frequencies are associated with distinct mental states.

There are many tracks available made strictly for hands-free orgasms (HFO). Search any porn streaming site, **Reddit** (HFO), **Soundgasm**, or **YouTube** for "HFO orgasm", or "tantric binaural".

Typically, **Alpha** (8 to 14 Hz) is related to a relaxed and calm state, often experienced during light meditation or day-dreaming. **Gamma** (30 to 100+ Hz) is associated with height-ened perception, cognitive processing, and possibly states of high-level awareness. Search audio and video streaming sites with the words "tantric", "arousal", or "sexual" for more intense frequencies. Responses to binaural beats and frequencies can also vary widely among individuals, influenced by factors like individual susceptibility, environmental conditions, and per-sonal preferences.

Electronica: The techno-digital genre, known for its pulsat-ing rhythms and immersive soundscapes, has the potential to make your prostate stomp, Hakken, and Shuffle. Its hypnotic beats and captivating melodies set a mood that can sync with the pace of prostate play, making an atmosphere conducive to heightened sensitivity. The wide range of sounds in elec-tronica stimulates your senses, enhances experiences, and cre-ates trance-like states. Its rhythmic patterns can complement movements and tactile sensations, raising pleasure levels.

Certain subgenres or tracks within electronica, particu-larly those with ambient or downtempo elements, possess a relaxing quality that aids in reducing inhibitions and stress during prostate play. This sense of relaxation can deepen the connection allowing for increased focus and enjoyment.

On the other side of this spectrum, hardcore and psychedelic house is the opposite of relaxation. But they can be helpful in getting lost in the frenetic energy of these sounds and snake-charm the prostate fluid from deep within while your prostate is getting hammered. Search any music streaming site or YouTube for "psychedelic trance, psytrance, or psy"; find tracks that interest you, then curate playlists for your play sessions.

While electronica can pump up the pleasure dial during anal play, its impact varies from person to person based on individual tastes. For example, a person from Detroit and someone from Berlin sitting next to each other in a bar are likely to have different reactions when a Kraftwerk song starts playing.

ASMR (Autonomous Sensory Meridian Response): This is a sensory experience where a tingling, often pleasant sensation starts on the scalp and travels down the neck and upper spine. It's triggered by specific auditory, visual, or tactile stimuli, such as whispers, tapping sounds, gentle touches, or even watching someone perform delicate tasks. People who experience ASMR often describe it as a calming, relaxing, and euphoric sensation that can bring a state of deep relaxation or even aid with sleep. ASMR can trigger arousal in different parts of the brain, offering a range of soothing sounds and mental visuals that aim to bring about this unique sensory response in individuals. Try the vanilla and erotic ASMR subcategories to find the best ways to tingle your mind and prostate. Search any porn streaming site, **Reddit, Soundgasm, Shibbydex,** or **YouTube** for "ASMR", "ASMR HFO", "Binaural Beats with ASMR". If you are good with media editing, you can create your own mixes for your play sessions.

Hypnosis: Audio designed for sexual enhancement via hypnosis taps into the subconscious mind to encourage heightened arousal, intimacy, and pleasure. These audio recordings often utilize suggestive language, guided imagery, and relaxation techniques to help individuals explore and enhance their sexual experiences. By addressing subconscious barriers, promoting relaxation, and offering positive affirmations, hypnosis audio strives to boost confidence, sensuality, and openness to new experiences.

It's important to note that the effectiveness of such audio varies among individuals and is recommended to approach these resources with an open mind and discretion, ensuring they align with your personal comfort levels and boundaries. You can find a hypnotist online as well and have them create a file just for you, based on your fetish and preferences.

JOI (Jerk off Instruction): Guided JOI audio offers interactive scenarios with a sexy voice leading you through a steamy journey, providing instructions and encouragement (or humiliation if you are into it) along the way. This is your chance to explore new fantasies, sensations, and desires. There are some really effective ones you can find online that focus on prostate play and cumming from anal (*see "Mindgasm" section*). Definitely check the ones that focus on anal first! Otherwise, search any porn streaming site, **Reddit** (JOI), **Soundgasm**, **Shibbydex**, or **YouTube**.

Audio Porn and Erotica Sources: This cums in many flavors! Moaning sex sounds, erotic stories, roleplay, sounds of BDSM, you name it. There is a flavor to suit every taste and fantasy. It works best when you find the fantasies you want to explore, and curate a titillating playlist before you start a prostate section. These stories work well with your imagination and can help you relax into your session.

Finding the right ones can require some research and patience. Visit porn streaming sites, **Reddit (Audiogonewild)**, **Soundgasm**, or **Shibbydex** for these. Many dominatrix content creators have files for purchase on **ManyVids**, **WarpMyMind.com**, or **HypnoTube**.

From guided masturbation tutorials to spicy erotic audio stories, there is something for everyone to enjoy while pleasuring your ears and your prostate. Remember, sound is powerful and should be included in your routines. It can greatly help tune your mind more into your body. You can find many of these genres on **YouTube**, **Vimeo**, **SoundCloud**, **Soundgasm**, **Reddit (r/gonewildaudio)**, **Patreon**, and other porn streaming sites. Bookmark your favorite ones or create your own curated mixes. Also, check the app stores (e.g., **Dipsea**, **Quinn**, **Emjoy**) for more customized and high-end paid options.

The Core of Exercise and Workouts

Studies show that physical exercise helps improve sex and orgasms. Heightened physical responses to exercise, such as elevated heart rate and breathing, bring an even greater physical response to sexual stimuli. The dilation of blood vessels during exercise improves circulation in the sexual organs, bringing more blood to the pelvic floor muscles and genital area; it also increases semen production. Several studies prove that regular physical activity keeps certain levels of hormones higher (such as dihydrotestosterone which is linked to orgasm frequency). Not only can regular physical exercise help with erections, but it can also help with achieving prostate orgasms.

More importantly, **a strong "core" will greatly improve your chances of becoming proficient in anal orgasms.** Your core muscles are the foundation of your body. And much like constructing a house, when it comes to anal play and kegel exercises, you need to start with a strong foundation. Your core is composed of the following parts:

- **Rector abdominis** – The "abs".
- **Gluteal muscles** – Your butt muscles, that are connected to your legs.
- **Erector spinae** – A muscle around the spine (how you stand up straight).
- **Obliques** – The sides of your torso (think twisting).

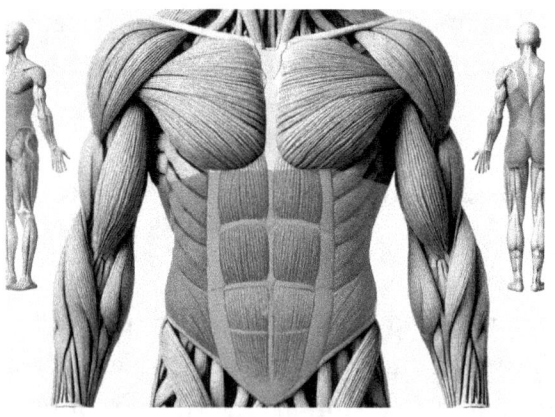

You don't need a six-pack like this to be strong—just a regular core routine for these areas.

When you are fully into your prostate sessions, many of these muscles will be activated. The goal is to increase your endurance and strength so you will be less tired during prolonged sessions. Exercise is the perfect way to improve sexual performance and pleasure.

If you are lucky, you might even have the elusive "coregasm"—an exercise-induced orgasm. Coregasms occur during physical activity when doing abdominal exercises. They are triggered by repeated contraction and fatigue of the core and pelvic muscles. While more common with cis women, the primary difference is that cis men ejaculate from coregasms and typically bypass an erection before ejaculation. A coregasm for men, however, is closer tied to a prostate orgasm versus a standard penile orgasm. Typically, coregasms occur when you are pushing past the point of fatigue to get through the few final reps of a workout.

Exercising tunes your body. Focus on workouts that target the pelvic floor so you can better stimulate yourself in more positions. This will also help you practice flexing and relaxing the muscles that achieve and control anal orgasms. Try squats, lunges, deadlifts, and other workouts that target your pelvic regions. Check out **musclewiki.com** for a free comprehensive library of targeted exercises.

Breathing

! **WARNING**: Breathwork can be a powerful practice, but it should be approached with care. If you have a medical condition such as heart issues, high blood pressure, respiratory problems, or a history of trauma, consult a healthcare professional before starting. Avoid prolonged breath retention or overexertion, as these can cause dizziness or discomfort. Always listen to your body, and if you feel lightheaded or unwell, stop immediately and return to normal breathing. This practice is not a substitute for medical advice or treatment. Proceed mindfully and responsibly.

For sexual arousal to occur, your body needs rich oxygen and increased circulation. Imagine your breath as a natural lube for your blood, easing its flow through your veins, capillaries, and heart, allowing your entire circulatory system to work smoothly and efficiently. It works like a natural Viagra. By using proper breathing techniques, you can lower cortisol levels and decrease the flow of prolactin in the body. This sparks a refreshed state that fuels heightened sexual energy.

Breathing is the ultimate arousal amplification technique. Moreover, a healthy mind efficiently produces more dopamine and oxytocin in your body, which act as supplements. Correct breathing balances nitric oxide in the blood, which helps muscles to relax, and widening of the blood vessels.

Close your eyes right now and take a second to tune into your breathing. Notice your breath. Is it slow and elongated? Is it fast and short? Are you in a sympathetic (fight or flight) or parasympathetic (calm and peaceful) state?

Focusing on your breathing will help you gain control over your body's automatic responses. **This leads to a more relaxed**

state of mind and lessens anxiety during sexual experiences. Additionally, mindful breathing can reduce stress and make prostate play more enjoyable.

Breathing is more than just an involuntary action—it's a powerful tool for enhancing focus, deepening sensations, and unlocking your body's full potential. By learning and practicing intentional breathing techniques, you can harness your breath to amplify pleasure, connect with your body, and stay grounded in the moment.

These breathing techniques explore various methods to elevate your sessions using the art of breath control. Again, think of the following section as a buffet of options, where you're free to select what suits you best. Each technique is different, and your task is to test and discover which resonates most with your comfort level. Repeat them for as long as you'd like:

(Before Play)

Breathwork before prostate play is helpful because it calms the mind and body, creating a more open state. Deep, intentional breathing activates the parasympathetic nervous system. This reduces tension and anxiety, allowing you to focus on sensations without distraction. Breathwork can also make it easier to engage and control your pelvic floor muscles. By combining mindful breathing with subtle muscle contractions, you can build a synergy between relaxation and stimulation even before you start stimulating your prostate. I recommend practicing breathwork for a minimum of 2 minutes beforehand, though it's even more effective when combined with a 10-minute meditation.

Belly and Circular Breathing Starter

1. On your back with your feet at hip-width distance, place your palms on your abdomen.
2. Rest your index fingers just above the pubic bone, and your thumbs just above your belly button. The tips of your index fingers and thumbs should touch one another so both hands together form a diamond pattern.
3. Breathe into your belly and pelvis for 5–20 breaths while observing the sensation in your body.
4. Do 3 seconds inhale, 3 seconds pause, and then 5 seconds exhale, with a 3-second pause before you repeat.

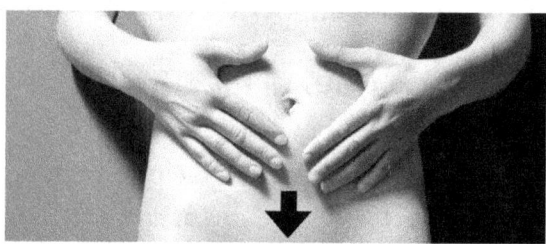

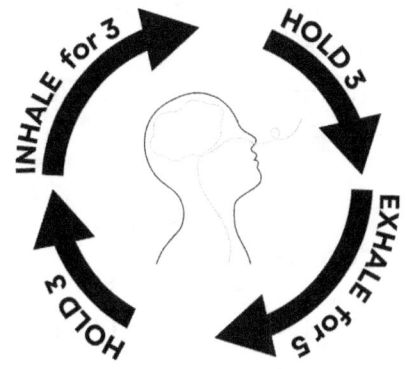

Sitting and Contracting Starter

1. Sit upright, eyes closed, and inhale slowly through the nose. Take a breath and imagine it coming up from the perineum area to the top of your head (pineal gland). Squeeze your pelvic floor muscles while inhaling. Hold your breath for 1-2 seconds.

2. Then, forcefully exhale through your nostrils while strongly contracting your abdomen. Pause for 2-3 seconds before you breathe again.

3. Take another slow inhale.

4. Focus fully on the inhales and exhales, feeling the pleasure and sexual energy build. Do this for 2-5 minutes.

Box Breathing

(My favorite one. Navy SEALs use it in high stress situations; and it's a great way for you to start a play session.)

1. Sitting, standing, or lying down, inhale deeply through your nose for 4 seconds.
2. Hold your breath for 4 seconds.
3. Exhale slowly through your mouth for 4 seconds.
4. Hold again for 4 seconds.

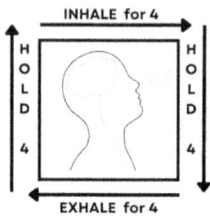

(During Play)

Don't forget to breathe through your nose during anal play. It is easy to forget to breathe, especially when you are riding a wave of pleasure. Holding your breath during sexual activity can limit the amount of new oxygen flowing into your system. Blood flow to your genital region is a natural part of the process of building an orgasm. And don't breathe short, fast (hyperventilating) breaths.

Natural slow breaths build arousal. Follow them with slow exhales. Make sure all breathing is done incorporating your diaphragm. It's all about breathing deeply through your stomach instead of taking shallow inhales and exhales through your chest.

Remember: **slow, controlled movements of the diaphragm and lower core muscles have a positive effect on producing anal orgasms.** Holding your breath during peak waves can prevent you from going over the critical edge.

Of course, everyone is different. Some people feel that when they get closer to orgasm, holding their breath for a short period will trigger an orgasm. Experiment with different breathing patterns to see what works for you. Keep mixing things up until you find the best technique.

I discovered that breathing slowly and shallowly while lightly tensing all my muscles worked best during my sessions. This technique helps me tune into my body's sensations and pinpoint the source of pleasure. For me, this spot is located in the pelvic floor area, radiating from deep within the perineum. Once you master proper breathing and identify your spot, you can adjust your muscle tension—either relaxing or increasing it—using your breath to control the levels of pleasure. This allows you to manage each stage of arousal, teasing out the sensations by either lowering or heightening them, prolonging the experience before anal orgasms fully take over.

When I'm in this state, I use breath techniques and muscle control to navigate the waves of pleasure and orgasms. When involuntary contractions begin and the orgasms take hold, I surrender to the sensations, slowing my breaths to savor every moment and extract an extra hit of pleasure. The key is to keep your breathing regulated at all times. Specialized breathwork not only enhances control but also extends the duration and intensity of the orgasmic waves.

> Deep diaphragmatic breathing with nipple play might just be the thing to help you crossover the edge when you are close to cumming.

First and foremost, learn how to contract and hold the two most important muscles, especially during breathwork. The perineum (the one you use to hold yourself from accidentally peeing) and the sphincter (the one you use to hold yourself from farting) are two of the most important areas when experimenting with anal orgasms (*see upcoming "Kegel" section for more details*).

Feel free to customize your experience with the following breath practices and techniques according to your preferences. Choose the one(s) that resonate with you and most align with your comfort level and personal situation. There's no need to try them all to achieve prostate orgasm mastery. Experiment, explore, and select what works best for you. The goal is to use these techniques to enhance and intensify sexual energy and orgasms during prostate play.

Qigong and Breathing

Qigong, pronounced "chi gong", has been around for thousands of years. It was developed in China as part of traditional Chinese medicine practice. The core of it involves using exercises to hone energy within the body, mind, and spirit, to improve and maintain health and well-being. Qigong contains both physical and psychological elements that involve the regulation of the mind, breath, body movement, and posture.

As you explore the basics of Qigong and release blockages in yourself, you become less self-absorbed, and more open to new experiences and more pleasure. This "chi" is a vital force in Taoism and is believed to be inherent in all things. Chi is considered to be the unimpeded circulation and a balance of negative and positive energy. When chi flows strongly within you, it becomes a healing and smoothing force that allows you to increase the sensitivity and awareness of the energy that flows throughout your body.

Simple Qigong Breathing Exercise

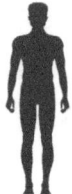

- **Find Your Position**: Stand with your feet shoulder-width apart, knees slightly bent, and arms relaxed at your sides. Or do this same variation lying down.
- **Inhale**: Breathe in deeply through your nose for 4 seconds, visualizing energy (positive or sexual) flowing into your body and filling your pelvic floor area.
- **Hold**: Hold your breath gently for 4 seconds, letting the energy settle and expand in your pelvic floor area and abdomen, squeezing the muscles in this area and smiling.
- **Exhale**: Breathe out slowly through your mouth for 6 seconds, imagining any tension or negative energy leaving your body.
- **Repeat**: Continue this cycle for 5–10 breaths, focusing on a smooth, steady rhythm and feeling a sense of calm and balance. Close your eyes for a deeper experience.
- You can also search for YouTube videos on "Anal Breathing Qigong" or "Qigong and sex" (specifically search for "Pelvic Pumping").

Orgasmic Breathing

- **Prepare:**
  - Close your eyes and begin to relax. Take 3 deep breaths to center yourself.
- **Engage Your Breath and Muscles:**
  - Inhale deeply through your nose for 5 seconds while clenching your sphincter (as if holding in a fart).
  - Exhale slowly for 5 seconds through your nose or mouth, releasing and pushing on your sphincter (as if letting out a long fart).
- **Focus on Sensations:**
  - Pay attention to the pleasurable sensations around your genitals, pelvic floor, and abdomen.
  - Feel the energy build and grow in this area as your body begins to open up.
- **Enhance the Experience:**
  - On each exhale, breathe out with a soft moan or sigh to intensify the sensations.
- **Practice and Expand:**
  - Complete 5-10 rounds of this breathing pattern.
  - With practice, notice twitching and minor waves of pleasure as they develop.
- **Repeat and Progress:**
  - Gradually increase the number of rounds over time.
  - With consistent effort, you may experience P-Gasms, or even a dry orgasm.

Double Helix Breath

Start by holding one hand over your stomach (diaphragm) and one over the middle of your chest. You are going to inhale from your nose quickly. Take the breath from your diaphragm for one quick half-second (hard breath). Do not exhale. Quickly inhale from your chest for one quick half-second (hard breath) then exhale deeply through your mouth for one second. Repeat the two quick inhale breaths through the nose, and release through your mouth, continuing for anywhere between 20-50 reps.

The longer you do this, the more intense the sensations will become. After you reach your limit, take one last breath, imagining it traveling from your anus to the crown of your heart. Do this slowly through the nose and hold it as long as you can. Release by breathing through the mouth slowly, imagining your breath pushing through your neck, chest, stomach and out your genitals.

Do this until you have mastered it comfortably. When you are ready to progress, make sure to squeeze the perineum on the first stomach breath, and hold it while simultaneously squeezing the sphincter muscle when you do the chest breath. Release with the exhales. During each of the short and long breaths, increase the intensity of the perineum and sphincter muscle squeezes. When you do your final long inhale, squeeze both, increasing as you get to the top of your breath. When you release your final breath, feel it travel through your genital area, and lightly squeeze the tip of your penis as if you feel it pulsating from an orgasm, or releasing cum. Ride the waves of convulsions.

For a guided experience, I highly recommend searching for YouTube videos featuring any of these breathwork techniques.

Additionally, visit **prostranal.com** for newly released and upcoming guided breathwork recordings designed specifically for prostate pleasure.

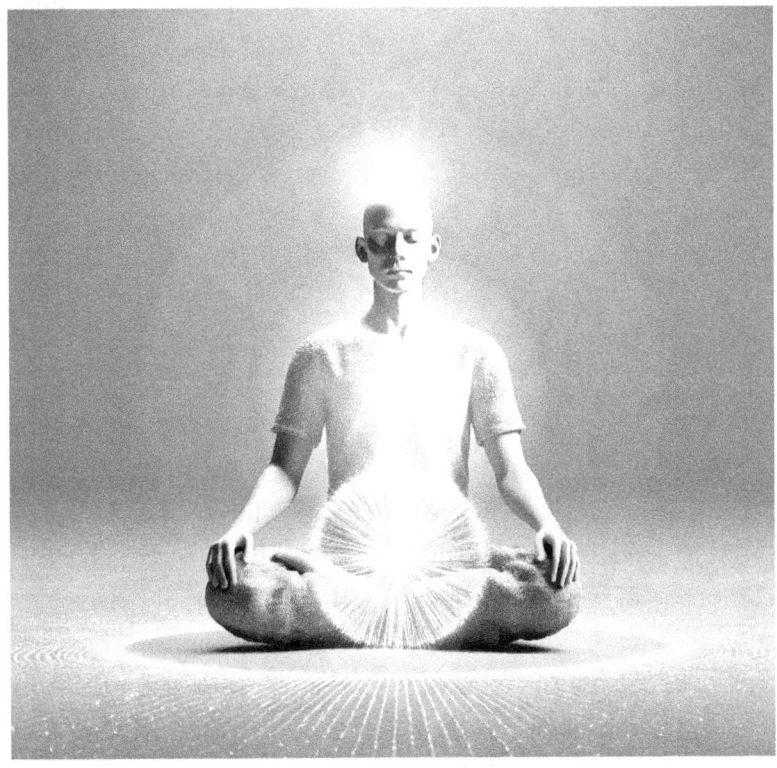

The breath and sex are intimately linked. To control your breath is to control your sexual energy, and to control your sexual energy is to control your life. — Mantak Chia

Nipple Play while Rubbing the Prostate

Stimulating the nipple and the surrounding areola for sexual pleasure is a technique known as "nipple play". Nipples, similar to the penis or clitoris, are composed of erectile tissue that stiffens and engorges upon arousal. The human nipple contains hundreds of sensitive nerve endings lying below the surface, making it a distinctly powerful erogenous zone.

Depending on one's nipple sensitivity, some can achieve a nipple orgasm without any genital stimulation. It is highly encouraged to experiment with your nipples during prostate play, since these nerves are connected to the same part of your brain that genital stimulation activates—the genital sensory cortex.

> Research shows that these nerves play a role in arousal and orgasm for all biological sexes.

When playing with your nipples, try different techniques: pulling, brushing lightly, milking, pinching, etc. It is best to combine this with soft touches around other erogenous zones such as your thighs, navel, chest, and neck. Some enthusiasts enjoy nipple pumps or using a vibrator on the nipples. You can even experiment with clit sucking toys as well.

If you are lucky, nipple play might just be the thing that sends your prostate over the edge.

Perineum Play

For one of your sessions, I highly recommend experimenting with the most underrated area of your body. The perineum, the area between the scrotum and the anus, plays a significant role in sexual pleasure, and can contribute to orgasms due to its dense network of nerves and proximity to other erogenous zones. You can stimulate the prostate gland externally by massaging the perineum. I call it the "front door" of your prostate. When stimulated indirectly through the perineum, powerful prostate orgasms can occur.

An orgasm achieved solely through perineum massage is known as a "perineum orgasm". When combined with the rhythmic activation and relaxation of the pelvic floor muscles, stimulation can significantly amplify the build-up and release of sexual pleasure. Intentional stimulation of the perineum often requires focus and mindfulness, which can heighten sensory awareness and intensify the orgasmic response. The combination of physical and mental engagement creates a pathway to deeper pleasure.

If you want to explore this, start with a gentle touch, then increase the pressure with firmer touches and rubbing. Place a couple of fingertips on the perineum and rub in a circular motion, stroking firmly through the skin. Firm pressure is the way to go over the edge. It can also be achieved with a vibrating wand, percussion gun, or hard anal toy (i.e., an njoy Pure Wand and kneading the area). Incorporate practicing pelvic floor contractions at the same time to build your arousal levels (*see "Toy and Kegel" section for techniques and more information*).

A little edging and penile play are also recommended. With practice, you could also achieve a very unique and intense blended anal orgasm. A good partner can help you achieve this.

Rewiring Your Body and Mind

Remember: No matter where you are on the path of sexual self-exploration, it is never too late to rewire your brain and physiology, and to start experimenting with different pathways of pleasure. Focus more on being relaxed and stop overthinking it. Anal orgasms are like the Pareto Principle: 80% of results come from 20% of the effort. Therefore, **anal orgasms are 80% mental and 20% physical**. Be aware of these two modes, knowing that your brain will be working harder than your prostate.

When you discover that your mind and ass can deliver powerful, body-shaking orgasms . . . there is no going back to the land of "normal". You will be forever changed and sexually happier. Rewiring yourself will make you more responsive to other forms of stimulation and pleasure: anus, prostate, frenulum, perineum, nipples, etc. You will also start to feel tingling pleasure in your pelvic area even when you are not playing with your prostate. You will feel other areas of your body increasing with sensitivity. You'll also discover another Pareto-like phenomenon: before exploring prostate play, you were likely experiencing only 20% of your potential pleasure.

However, **it takes time to build these new pathways for pleasure**. Rewiring occurs when you activate the neural circuitry in your brain. The goal is to understand the feeling of orgasm in the brain, instead of only in the penis. This usually means avoiding penis stimulation while focusing on prostate play. And this can be challenging for many. Once again, you need to be a warrior on this prostate journey. Your job is guarding the sperm bank—do not rob your own vault!

Learning to become responsive to non-penile stimulation requires your body to go through a transformation. **It's like unlocking a hidden level in a video game**—you've been playing the same way for years, but once you discover a new approach, a whole new experience opens up. You become more aware of sensations in your body, specifically the pelvic and genital areas. Your erections also become stronger as you awaken your urogenital galaxy. Best of all, this increase in sexual sensitivity leads to spontaneous positive stimulus and non-ejaculatory orgasms. Soon you are able to control and create various types of orgasms: dry, wet, Super O, energy, etc.

Although it may sound complex, rewiring is actually a simple process. It is the act of awakening your ass and prostate nerve pathways. It doesn't change who you are or subtract from your sexuality. It just adds to your pleasure skill set. It also helps you recognize the physical and emotional layers of anal play.

Eventually, the pleasure rewards from multiple prostate orgasms become much greater than penile orgasms. And the more you rewire yourself, the deeper and more intense your pleasure becomes. Orgasm is typically thought to be concentrated in the genital area. However, your orgasm occurs throughout your entire body (and mind). You learn that moving your focus away from one area allows you to expand your limits of sexual pleasure and open yourself to a new path of sexual exploration. You also learn that sexual energy and pleasure are connected throughout the body, as you unlock these pleasure pathways and channels.

What I've discovered during sex with my partner is that prostate play takes everything to a whole new level once you learn to rewire. When I wear a plug or use an Aneros toy during sex (or even if I don't), I start off already experiencing P-Gasms and dry orgasms—my body becomes this incredible vessel for pleasure. It's like a singularity of sensation, building and intensifying with every moment. Everything gets amplified: my erection, my desire, my creativity—it's like turning the pleasure dial to maximum. I'm no longer focused on chasing a penile orgasm; instead, I'm lost in a trance, yet fully present, as infinite waves of pleasure surge through me like tornadoes of orgasms touching down across my entire body. Sex was fun before I explored prostate play, but now it's an utterly mind-blowing experience.

Solo play is the best place to practice and learn this psychological redirection of your erogenous zones. It is an essential training ground for exploring new sensations. Rather than solely focusing on your penis as the primary sexual organ, you learn how to shift your attention from the base of your penis toward the perineum and ultimately to the external and internal anal area. By exploring these sensitive nerve regions of the anus and prostate, you can experience faster anal orgasms. It's crucial to relax and allow yourself to embrace these sensations naturally and slowly.

Traditionally, penis owners (specifically individuals assigned male at birth) do not consider their anal area as an erotic erogenous zone. However, you can change this thinking by changing your mindset and recognizing the potential for erotic pleasure. Over time and with practice, it's possible to rewire your conditioned mind, and redirect your pleasure onto these new erogenous pathways. I often say that it's like being a teenager all over again. Once you start discovering how to unlock pleasure in these areas, you might find yourself staying home more often, "busy" behind closed doors for a while.

Rewiring the prostate involves practice with massaging new regions of your body. It's an adventure worthy of Indiana Jones, full of discovery and bold exploration. You are going to have to map out these areas to bring them to light. In time, you will fully enjoy, and even reach climax, solely through anal and prostate stimulation, without completely abandoning the pleasures associated with the penis. **It's important to remember that this journey is a gradual process, and not something that can be achieved overnight.** The goal is to mindfully connect the prostate and orgasm, creating positive sensory feedback loops.

Once you learn to rewire, most likely you will move into A-less—a term created to reference prostate pleasure without having an Aneros toy (a brand of prostate massager) inserted during prostate play. A-less means "Aneros Less" or "without an Aneros". A-less is a mind orgasm that can induce prostate pleasure and orgasm using only breathing, concentration, and contractions. Once you master anal play, it gets much easier to achieve A-less orgasms. Best of all, you can orgasm without all the prep and cleanup required for a traditional prostate session.

There's also an online series called *Mindgasm*. It provides training on how to achieve these types of orgasms. This program helped me rewire to achieve consistent and stronger anal orgasms. I cannot recommend it enough. (*See "Mindgasm Versus A-Less" section for details.*)

Semen Retention

Semen contains sperm cells, water, enzymes, proteins, fructose, citric acid, zinc, potassium, calcium, magnesium, sodium, vitamin C, lactic acid, urea, uric acid, nitrogen, creatine, cholesterol, prostaglandins, and various hormones such as testosterone and oxytocin.

Semen or sperm retention is the sexual act of not ejaculating. This topic creates some disagreement in the prostrainer community. In short, semen retention requires that you to not ejaculate for anywhere from 3 days to weeks. This will naturally increase your sex drive and make you more sensitive to anal play, as well as other sources of stimuli. One study saw a 145% increase in testosterone in one week of not ejaculating (masturbating).

This holding back allows the prostate to feel swollen, hence easier to stimulate. Many believe you should hold off for as long as possible between ejaculatory releases. This is a bit old school and similar to Tantra and Taoist sexual practices. Some prefer "edging" over pure abstinence. This is when you masturbate and get close to orgasm, stopping before climaxing; repeating over and over so you build up intense sexual energy. I prefer this method and then go straight to prostate play.

One method you might want to try is to slowly reduce/trickle-down your ejaculatory orgasm and penis play over time. For example, slowly play with your cock less and less over a few weeks. Incorporate more anal play over the same time. Cum from your penis every other day, then go to once a week, etc. This slowly gets your body to associate orgasms and prostate play with sexual pleasure.

On the other side of the fence, consistent anal play is important to rewire your sexual programming. The more stimulation, the better you get at building on your skills. But similarly to going to the gym, you can get sore and lose gains if you push yourself too hard. And your anal/prostate sensitivity gradually diminishes.

Realistically, you can achieve prostate orgasms anytime the mood arrives. And as you progress, you will be able to have strong anal orgasms even after penile orgasms.

Constant exploration and experimentation help rewire your brain more effectively for pleasure beyond just your penis. And remember, urologists recommend frequent ejaculations; research has shown that flushing your prostate helps reduce the likelihood of prostate issues.

If you want a perfect compromise for semen retention (and you are brave enough) try swallowing your cum after ejaculation. You could say it's a form of recycling energy. Supposedly, it is good for your immune system—if you can stomach the taste. In Ancient Greece, semen was considered a source of wisdom and masculinity. Certain Amazonian tribes historically believed semen played a role in strengthening warriors and connecting them with spiritual forces. Various Pacific Island cultures have rituals where drinking bodily fluids (including semen) symbolizes power transfer, initiation, and bonding.

A positive feedback loop in sexual arousal is like a self-reinforcing pleasure cycle— where stimulation, sensation, arousal, orgasm continuously amplify each other. When the mind and body are in sync, even tiny sensations can trigger a domino effect of pleasure, making arousal more intense and prolonged—continuously repeating and building upon itself.

CHAPTER 6
PELVIC FLOOR MUSCLE EXERCISES

(AKA KEGELS)

Overview

- Kegels activate the prostate and key nerve pathways for deeper pleasure.
- Learn the PAT method to strengthen pelvic floor muscles and enhance sensations.
- Discover techniques, breathing integration, and other muscle engagement tips.
- Time to get active—this chapter is your first prostate workout!

As mentioned in an earlier chapter, learning to do kegels helps stimulate and awaken the prostate, pudendal, perineal nerves, and associated muscles. These voluntary contractions are essential to achieving anal orgasms. As an analogy, **think of the pelvic floor muscles as you would a bicep when you're at the gym**. Imagine your goal one day is to squeeze a walnut with your bicep and break it open. Now, if you've never been to the gym, your bicep is likely weak. It is going to take some time to be able to reach this goal.

You are going to have to dedicate time to practice your pelvic floor muscle exercises. Fortunately, they are easy to do and can be done anywhere, even with clothes on. If you've ever stopped your urine flow midstream, or consciously held in a fart (gas), then you have already done a kegel. There are two types of kegels. You are either "pushing out" or "clenching in". **A regular kegel is clenching (the same muscle/feeling you have when holding in your urine and/or fart). A reverse kegel is pushing (the same feeling when you are urinating and/or pooping).**

Consistency forms the strength of your pelvic muscles. Build your disciplined schedule and do it anywhere you can. Much like the gym, these are muscles that need to be trained. Just as it takes time to build new neuropaths for pleasure, it will take time to condition your pelvic floor area.

When you learn to kegel correctly, something will begin changing inside of you. For instance, a warm and tingling sensation right at the base of the penis will form that you have never felt before. Or the scrotum area will feel like it is connected to the tip of the penis (This is called the frenulum, the underside of the tip. It is the most sensitive part.). A newfound sexual power awakens within you, unlocking a heightened sense of awareness and ecstasy beyond anything you've ever imagined.

Kegel exercises have been around for centuries. The kegel is named for its inventor, Dr. Arnold Kegel, a gynecologist in the early-to mid-20th century, who researched and developed pelvic floor exercises. Prior to him, there were many ancient Asian cultures that practiced these exercises in yoga and other spiritual rituals.

In the following sections, I will provide various kegel exercises to stimulate your prostate. And I highly recommend you alternate the clenching and pushing in the rhythmic variations during these exercises. Remember the staircase vertical line? You want to create new experience and techniques, especially here!

While practicing these exercises, you will learn to create powerful voluntary and involuntary contractions, as well as build stronger pelvic floor muscles. Your pleasure sensations will either grow and increase, or they may stay the same and plateau at times. The goal is to practice, practice, and practice. Over time, these waves of pleasure will intensify as you discover what your body truly craves. **The goal is to transform voluntary contractions into effortless, involuntary ones.**

In the following group of exercises, we are going to practice with various muscle groups. You can practice anywhere, in a chair, standing, or lying down. As a beginner, I recommend lying down and creating a relaxed environment, as mentioned in the earlier chapter, Relaxation Techniques. The better the setting, the better the results. I also recommend doing one round of relaxation breathing before you begin.

But first, let's learn the **PAT** method:

- **P**-Muscle: holds pee functions.
- **A**-Muscle: holds ass functions (e.g., gas, rectum from defecating).
- **T**-Muscle: the tip, the tingly part that you feel at the tip of your penis before you cum.

> An easy way to remember the PAT muscles is: **P** stands for the **penis muscle**, **A** for the **ass muscle**, and **T** for the **tip muscle**.

The A-Muscle is easy to pinpoint. Insert a small toy, anal plug, or finger and you can rock it back and forth with kegel contractions (push or pull) using your sphincter and pubo-coccygeus muscle (*see diagram*). On the other hand, your P-muscle and T-Muscle can be tricky to find and challenging to control.

Let's start with the P-Muscle. Find it the next time you urinate. Press your finger on the perineum (the lined area between your scrotum and anus) and stop midstream while urinating. You should be able to feel it pulse under your finger and feel the muscle area contracted. Begin to urinate again and stop. This time, instead of using your finger, use your whole palm to feel the muscle areas—mostly the ischiocavernosus and some bulbospongiosus muscles (*see diagram*)—being used to hold back your pee. This is the feeling you should have when you practice your kegel P-Muscle contractions.

Now, grab your flaccid cock and stretch it by the head. Stretch as far and long you can—but not to the point of any pain. Next, flex your P-Muscle slowly and gently. Your cock should start to feel like it is getting shorter (retracting) as you flex your P-Muscle. Increase the strength of your flexes. A strong flex should be felt in the perineum and testes area (since you are using the bulbospongiosus muscle). Close your eyes and really imagine and feel these muscles in the diagram being used. Alternate between your A-muscle and P-Muscle when doing this so you can feel the differences and similarities of muscles. This is the best way to fine-tune the use of these muscles.

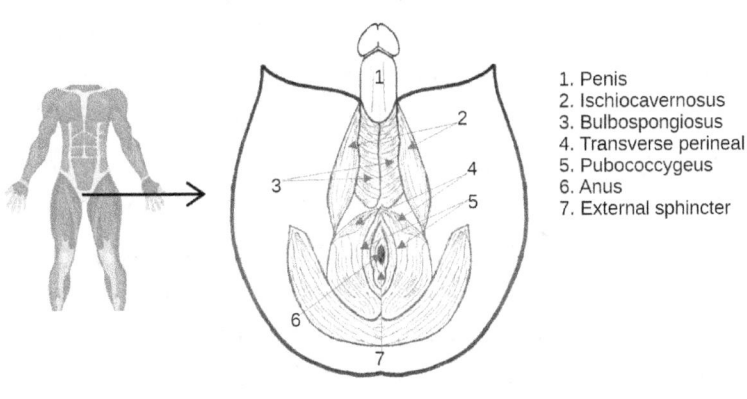

1. Penis
2. Ischiocavernosus
3. Bulbospongiosus
4. Transverse perineal
5. Pubococcygeus
6. Anus
7. External sphincter

All the muscles and key areas used in the PAT Method.

Bulbopongiosus muscle (BC) – Located at the base of the penis shaft, it helps regulate blood flow into your penis, creating erections and controlling ejaculation.

Pubococcygeus muscle (PC) – Forms at the top of the pubic bone and goes all the way to the tailbone. You feel it contract during orgasm. It is the muscle that will help you learn to have multiple orgasms.

Ischiocavernous muscle (IC) – Next to the BC muscle, this one keeps your penis hard and is the one you use when you move your dick around without your hand.

For the T-Muscle, you gently flex the ischiocavernosus and pubococcygeus muscles, primarily the levator prostatae—a section of the pubococcygeus made up of medial and ventral fibers that insert into the tissue in front of the anus; this section connects to and supports the prostate gland. These muscles run along the sides of the base of your penis. That said, the T-Muscle is mostly a "mental muscle" that you feel in the head of the penis. You also feel it around the base of your shaft and pubic area. If you struggle with finding it, just imagine there is a muscle in the tip of your penis that you're flexing (i.e., try to visualize the lips of your penis trying to touch). The best way to find it is by doing a long P-Muscle hold (15 seconds if you can) then releasing slowly and trying to locate your T-Muscle. You should be able to hold a T-Muscle flex and cause involuntary contractions. You'll notice that when the P-Muscle contracts, it is more difficult to contract the T-Muscle at the same time. If you still can't find the T-Muscle, try these techniques:

- Imagine you are trying to pull your penis head under your scrotum
- Flex the muscle that connects the base where your pubic hair starts (just below the belly button, use a finger there if you need help to contract it).
- Lightly visualize that you are pushing out pee or (cum) and using a very light P-Muscle and A-Muscle contraction, imagining the pee or (cum) coming from that area and heading toward your penis head.
- Look down at your penis and see the vein that runs from the base to the head. Imagine you are pushing out a small pea-shaped object from end to end. Imagine it getting ever so slightly stuck at the tip and you are trying to push it out with light contractions.

These are the three primary pelvic floor muscles that you will be practicing with in the next section. Do each of these introductory warm-ups in your bed, while on your back, in a comfortable environment before moving on to more advanced pelvic floor exercises. Remember to keep breathing deeply and slowly! Sensations will grow and increase. Over time, your technique will improve, and it will increase the contractions and intensity.

> **Tip**: For best results, do pelvic floor exercises with a toy inside you to activate pleasure. Pushing the toy inside while pushing out with the pelvic floor muscles will eventually bring arousal. Building up tension this way helps force muscle contractions. Push harder and harder with both the toy and the

muscles as you become more experienced. With vibrating toys, try squeezing your kegel following your toy vibration pattern.

What To Feel For

If you are new to kegels, it will feel like you are in a dark room looking for a light switch, asking yourself, "What should I be feeling for?" At first, expect nothing and have no expectations for outcomes. This is the best way to approach pelvic floor exercises. Rest in this space and let the feelings come to you. In time, you will begin to feel what some call "prostate tickles". Get the mental and physical tension to build. Try finding the faint sensations when you do your kegels, focusing on them, and allowing them to grow. It is about relaxing and letting the feelings build. Early on, there may be some days where you cannot find the tickle, and some days that you can. So be patient. It will require you to focus away from your traditional penis orgasm wiring. You are looking for the tingling-static electricity sensations hidden deeper within your nervous system and prostate area.

Repeat this search over and over, unlocking the secrets of your body. Eventually, you will find the tingling and buzzing sensations faster, stronger, and longer. Like a runner, you need to build skill and stamina. Timing and refinement are everything with kegels. Your ability to hold kegels longer will help, as well as being able to master the ranges of light to hard kegel holds. If you keep practicing, you will be able go the distance and get involuntarily contractions. This is the way to become wrapped in orgasmic bliss.

The following warm-up routines will greatly assist you in unlocking this experience.

P-Muscle Warm Up

Take several deep breaths, then return to natural breathing. Relax your stomach and buttocks so you do not use these muscle groups. Slightly spread your legs apart. Consciously and slowly squeeze your P-Muscle, as if you are trying to stop urinating midstream. Build slowly and hold for 5 to 10 seconds. Release gently and slowly.

Start the next one right afterward. Increase the intensity each time. For example, start your first one at a low-intensity level, then a moderate squeeze. Then do your last one or two at the hardest/high squeeze level. Focus on relaxing the rest of your body as much as you can while practicing these techniques.

Do 5 rounds of 5 P-Muscle warm-ups and rest for 30-60 seconds. Practice as many rounds as you can until you fatigue or master the technique. Aim for doing this for 5-10 minutes each day for one week. Repeat 5 times.

> Think of these muscles as an elevator going up and down. As you contract and squeeze them, the elevator slowly rises to the top. As you gently release the tension in your muscles, imagine the elevator returning to ground level.

A-Muscle Warm Up

Similar to the P-Muscle . . . take several deep breaths, then return to natural breathing. Relax your stomach and buttocks so you do not use these muscle groups. Slightly spread your legs apart. Consciously and slowly squeeze your A-Muscle, as if you are trying to stop from passing gas or holding a bowel movement. Build slowly and hold for 5 to 10 seconds. Release gently and slowly. Start the next one right afterward. Increase the intensity each time—for example, start your first one at a low-intensity level, then a moderate squeeze, and then do your last one or two at the hardest/high squeeze level. Focus on relaxing the rest of your body as much as you can while practicing these techniques.

Do 5 rounds of 5 A-Muscle warm-ups, and rest for 30-60 seconds. Practice as many rounds as you can until you fatigue or master the technique. Aim to do this for 5-10 minutes each day for one week, after your P-Muscle warm-ups.

Repeat 5 times. Practice this routine after your P-Muscle warm-ups. Do them every day for one week.

All Together Now

Once you've mastered both, practice squeezing your P-Muscle and A-Muscle at the same time. This tightening of your pelvic floor muscles will be more intense and challenging. Take your time, and close your eyes to concentrate, slowing down your breathing with deep breaths from your diaphragm.

Again, relax your stomach and buttocks. You don't want to exercise those muscle groups. Slightly spread your legs apart. Consciously squeeze your P-Muscle and A-Muscle at the same time. Build slowly and hold for 5 to 10 seconds. Release gently and slowly.

Increase the intensity each time. Start your first one at a low-intensity level, then a moderate squeeze, and do your last one or two at the hardest/high squeeze level.

Do 5 rounds *without* resting in between this exercise. Go for as many rounds as you can until you fatigue. Aim for doing this 10-20 minutes a day for one week.

Remember to relax the rest of your body as much as possible. Don't be surprised if you start to feel strong arousal sensations and contractions as you improve your focus and technique. If you experience contractions, don't resist them or let them disrupt your clenching. Be like a bull rider! Always ride the waves of pleasure for as long as you can.

Reverse Kegels

Reverse kegels are the inverse of the PAT Method. You push out and hold like you are peeing and push out like you are pooping. Reverse kegels are just as important as regular kegels.

I suggest standing straight up and tall, draw a full diaphragm inhale breath, one that reaches the very bottom of your torso. Let this breath put pressure into your pelvic region, then carefully and slowly squeeze your lower abs as you exhale and push the breath down, like trying to push pee out on an empty bladder. On your next breath, do the same thing — but this time, as you exhale, push the breath down so you feel like you are pushing a poop/fart out of your stomach. Be careful when you first try these reverse kegels. It could feel tight and tense. Do not continue if it hurts or feels like you are going to have a bowel or bladder movement. On a scale of soft, moderate and hard clenching, try to clench your muscles softly when you start reverse kegels. Aim for a low to mid-level contraction. Once you get the feel for it, use the aforementioned P and A warm-ups with only reverse kegels.

Practice this Reverse kegel using the P and A warm-ups you learned earlier every day for a week. It is a good idea to also do a round of regular P and A warm-ups right after your reverse kegel routine so you can feel and learn the differences in sensations.

Other Areas "Nearby Pelvic Floor Region Exercises"

The road to heaven is paved with good contractions.

After you mastered the basics of the PAT Method, feel free to incorporate these extra delights into your pelvic routine or anal play. The nearby pelvic floor areas will still slightly engage the P- and A-Muscles. However, do not let the P-Muscles and A-Muscles become the focus in these exercises.

T-Muscle Practice

This will be the most challenging muscle to master. But **the T-Muscle is the key to strong prostate orgasms, and the secret to your success.** *(Reread and use the suggestions discussed earlier in this chapter about the T-Muscle. Trust me! It's worth* *learning this.)*

One of the best practices is to imagine the lips of your penis trying to touch, opening and closing ever so lightly. Try contracting that area and the tip. Do this lightly and tune into the subtle sensations when training this area. You will still slightly engage the P- and A-Muscles, but do not let them take over when focusing on the T-Muscle.

Hold it for as long as you can (preferably with a toy stimulating your prostate). You should start to feel involuntary contractions over time. Don't be shy about pressing your fingers around the tip area to find it as you experiment with contractions.

Here is a good practice T-Muscle routine to do first:

- Take several deep breaths, then return to natural breathing. Lightly squeeze your T-Muscle every 1-3 seconds and then release for 1-3 seconds. Continue doing these for 2-5 minutes. You can sync it to your breathing if you like. Or just breathe naturally.

When you feel comfortable with the first routine, do this T-Muscle one next:

- Take several deep breaths, then return to natural breathing. Squeeze your A-Muscle to 50% of your full-strength clench. Hold for 30-60 seconds. Relax the rest of your body as much as possible. Keep holding and lightly squeeze your T-Muscle. After a while, you will notice the energy and pleasure move up to your penis head. Pay close attention and imagine it like a thermometer of pleasure moving up your ure-thra. Soon you will feel your penis head throbbing and filling with tingly sensations. If you experience contractions, don't resist them or let them disrupt your clenching. Ride the waves of pleasure for as long as you can.

Feel free to play with different variations of this. For example, start with a P-Muscle squeeze instead of an A-Muscle squeeze. Or squeeze all three. Once you've mastered the T-Muscle, you can experiment with unlimited variations. For example, squeeze and pulse rhythmically instead of holding it steady (i.e., instead of imagining the lips on your penis trying to seal a kiss, imagine the lips opening and closing like a goldfish's mouth). As you get better at using the T-Muscle, focus on the spot just above your penis root and the line of your pubic hair. You can press down with your finger above the pubic bone to find it or activate it if you'd like. Once you find it, use your imagination to control this area and go a little higher every time in the direction of your belly button. The higher the spot (not more than 1.5 inches), the more intense the orgasm.

Find a good middle ground for your T-Muscle squeeze, just between too weak and too strong. It comes down to being able to flex much smaller areas of the pelvic floor muscles with pinpoint accuracy. You are learning to separate the muscles here, and as you get better at this, you will find deeper orgasmic sensations and longer sets of contractions. It is crucial not to disrupt the flow of pleasure by clenching other muscles, breathing too rapidly, losing mental focus, or feeling the urge to touch your penis. When the contractions subside, shift your attention to slow, deep diaphragmatic nose breathing, and focus on the lingering sensations and other parts of your body for continued pleasure. This helps reset your body, paving the way for the next wave of contractions as you resume your clenching exercises.

Tail Bone

Similar to the P-Muscle and A-Muscle exercises . . . relax your stomach and buttocks so you do not use these muscle groups. Take several deep breaths, then return to natural breathing. Slightly spread your legs apart. Consciously and slowly squeeze your tailbone muscle by imagining squeezing the skin between the top of your butt crack. Or imagine the tip of your tailbone radiating pleasure and vibrating. Then focus on locking into that while gently squeezing your core and butt cheeks. You should now start to feel the same tingly pleasure you felt from your PAT exercises. The difference is that the sensations and contractions now radiate from behind.

Build slowly and hold for 5 to 10 seconds. Release gently and slowly. Start the next one right afterward. Increase the intensity each time. For example, start your first one at a low-intensity level, then a moderate squeeze. Do your last one or two at the hardest/high squeeze level.

Do 5 rounds of 5 tailbone muscle warm-ups, then rest for 30-60 seconds. Practice as many rounds as you can until you fatigue or master the technique. Aim for doing this 5 minutes a day.

Feel free to experiment with different variations by incorporating squeezes from other muscles.

Scrotum Rolls

Some call these "testicle lifters". The best way to start is to imagine rolling and folding the skin of your scrotum. You will be engaging your cremaster muscles that will induce extra tingly sensations. The cremaster muscle is a series of tiny fibers that run in the spermatic cord to the testicles all the way from the groin to the side of your penis. You have two testes, two cords, two cremaster muscles that can act like a puppet master of pleasure.

You can pulse and create waves of pleasure by relaxing the scrotum muscle, then tightening it. It also can be done by imagining you are ever so slightly lifting your balls up and down, similar to doing dumbbell shrugs for your traps. You want to feel the pleasure and sensations coming from the center of the scrotum, right where the little cavity forms below the base of your penis. It will be tempting to tighten your P-Muscle but try to make the contraction come from the scrotum. Practice for 15-30 seconds and rest. Try for 5 rounds. This is a bonus pleasure delight that you can add anytime with your PAT kegels.

CHAPTER 7

MORE PELVIC FLOOR MUSCLE TECHNIQUES WITH BREATHWORK

Overview

- Take your pelvic floor training to the next level with advanced PAT Method techniques.
- Strengthen control and intensify sensations with more challenging breath and muscle engagement.
- Get so good at pelvic floor control you could sign a check with your sphincter while holding your breath for minutes.

Now that you better understand the basics, from here on out it is best to experiment with a toy inserted for maximum pleasure and sensitivity for the following activities. I recommend using a prostate toy or butt plug during practice sessions. This enhances sensation and helps fine-tune your clenching for greater pleasure.

Just remember, like other muscle groups, **it can take between 1 to 4 weeks to start seeing improvement in your**

control and function. Keep in mind that progress can happen more quickly depending on your training routine and how closely you follow the guidance in this book.

When you get closer to the edge of dry, wet, and Super-Os during anal play, take all the techniques mentioned and create your own explosive combination. I usually prefer doing a P-Muscle and A-Muscle high-level squeeze, then incorporate scrotum rolls, until I explode. Another technique I use is 3 to 5 seconds of reverse kegel ("pushing out"), then 3 to 5 seconds of regular kegel squeezing (both P and A). When the feeling of cumming gets close to the peak, I incorporate T-Muscle squeezing and contracting to reach my wet orgasm.

Incorporate this with rhythmic hip movements and core squeezing with deep breaths, and you will erupt. Look for a mild spasm, quivers, and a pulsing feeling. Lock on when you feel them and increase the sensations by squeezing harder.

Remember to keep breathing as you hold the squeeze patterns. Focus on *firm* but not hard pressure to the top of the prostate where the ampulla and seminal vesicles meet the prostate. Also, alternate moderate to light contractions, gently thrusting down. When you start to feel the P-Waves, relax into them instead of tensing up everywhere.

By massaging the prostate and learning pelvic floor muscle techniques, you will reach new levels of mastery. Be assured that once this alignment occurs, you will never want to go back. It will set you on a path of deeper exploration and wonder. With enough practice, the resulting anal and penile orgasm releases will become non-refractory type orgasms. There will be no cool-down or recovery period, and you get to experience multiple orgasms, possibly for hours.

When I was younger, I could easily have three penile

ejaculatory orgasms in a day, but as I got older, that became impossible—until I discovered prostate orgasms. Now, after a great prostate session, I often find myself craving three "hands-on" penile orgasms in a single day. It's like reclaiming the vitality and energy I thought was long gone with my youth. This is a common theme you'll hear across the pros-trainer community. And why so many older enthusiasts freely share their stories. Awakening your prostate is like finding the fountain of youth.

Now that you've mastered the PAT Method, I strongly encourage you to take it to the next level by exploring these more advanced and challenging techniques. You can try these exercises lying down or sitting.

Rhythm Builder Method

Lightly squeeze your A-Muscle, and let go of it. Then squeeze the P-Muscle, and let go of it. Then squeeze the T-Muscle, and let go of it. Keep repeating to build the squeeze stronger after each set. Slowly increase the speed and keep the rhythm. Follow your breath with the movements. See how long and fast you can go. When you can't go any faster or tire out, hold all three muscles taking in a deep belly breath. Hold for at least 10 seconds (longer is better but use caution and do not pass out). Tighten your abdominal muscles as well. When you are ready, release the breath for a long as you can while doing a reverse kegel, pushing all three muscles out at the same time with your breath.

My "Rolling Up and Down" Method

Take a deep diaphragm breath and do a moderate squeeze of P-Muscle and A-Muscle, holding for 3 seconds. Release and do a moderate reverse kegel for 3 seconds. Keep doing this for a minute, then increase to a high level of squeezing, and getting them down to 1 second each. You can match your breath to the squeezing. As you grow this sexual energy, you should start to feel it turn into a wave motion and eventually it will be just quick pulsating back and forth.

OPTION: Do this with a metronome playing. Use one that increases speed to help you follow along.

In and Out Method

Breathe deeply and slowly contract your P-Muscle and A-Muscle to a light level as you inhale—do not hold your breath at the top. As you exhale, gently perform a reverse kegel at a very light level, focusing on relaxing and expanding the same areas. Continue this cycle, gradually increasing the intensity of your contractions during the inhale, while keeping your reverse kegels at a moderate level during the exhale. As you begin to feel involuntary contractions or waves of sensation, follow them—pulse and contract your P-Muscle, A-Muscle and T-Muscle in sync with your body's rhythm. Let the contractions build naturally until you reach a plateau, then gently reset and repeat the cycle.

Finding More Breathwork Techniques

There are many books that provide breathing exercises you can explore, and incorporate during your prostate sessions, if you are so inclined. They are often rooted in Tao, Tantra, and other Eastern practices. From "Cobra breath" to "Fire Breath", there are many breathing techniques that work perfectly with prostate play—especially when using a prostate toy. I recommend visiting the Internet Archive library and searching for these topics. One book in particular I highly recommend is *The Alchemy Of Sexual Energy Connecting to the Universe from Within* by Mantak Chia. Also, *Urban Tantra* by Barbara Carrellas.

Breathwork is a powerful method for relaxing the nervous system, stimulating circulation and arousal, and generating more energy. Learning a meditation practice and breathing techniques are essential for advanced prostate pleasure. Do not underestimate these practices. They are the gateway to incredible orgasms. Shallow and unstructured breathing will make it more difficult to build up your levels of arousal.

I highly recommend exploring holotropic breathing. **It is a powerful breathwork practice designed to achieve altered states of consciousness for healing, self-exploration, and personal growth.** Holotropic breathing is valued for its ability to promote emotional release, self-awareness, and spiritual connection. It is often used to address unresolved traumas, gain clarity, and achieve personal transformation. However, the practice can be intense and is not suitable for everyone. Individuals with medical conditions such as heart issues, epilepsy, pregnancy, or severe mental health challenges should avoid it. Much like an Ayahuasca ceremony, it can be an intense, almost psychedelic experience, unlocking deep emotions and even resurfacing buried memories.

It's essential to practice holotropic breathing under the guidance of a certified facilitator in a safe environment to have a happy and safe experience.

CHAPTER 8

LEVELS OF AROUSAL

Overview

- Explore the 10 levels of arousal and how they build toward orgasm.
- Understand orgasm styles and why everyone's is unique.
- This chapter shows how orgasms are like elevator rides—everyone goes up and down differently.

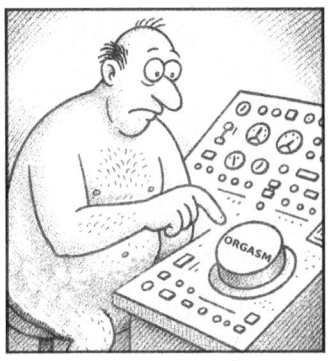

Carl had reached Level 9 of the Pleasure Protocol. The final stage was to become the button.

The following graph shows a standard Super-O, or intense anal orgasm progression with continual stimulation of the prostate. As you can see, the pleasure peak is usually a steady rise with peaks of P-Waves and smaller anal orgasms at different intervals. It is not uncommon that post-orgasm brings some anal soreness and discomfort, depending on how long your session lasts. If you are feeling this discomfort, stopping play for a few minutes can easily reduce soreness and help get you back on the arousal highway. And always follow the golden rule of prostate play: **never continue when you feel pain!**

Everyone's arousal levels will be different. Some individuals have multiple Super-Os where their orgasms can last from anywhere between a few minutes to an hour. The more you explore, the better you will understand your range and limitations.

For me, I usually have P-Waves and an anal orgasm (moderate level) within 15-30 seconds. The pleasure level for both increases every five minutes. My Super-O or final anal (wet) orgasm occurs between 20-45 minutes. Then I reach a point where my prostate becomes a little sore, and I stop. I've had two-hour sessions with two to three Super-Os, though they are rare.

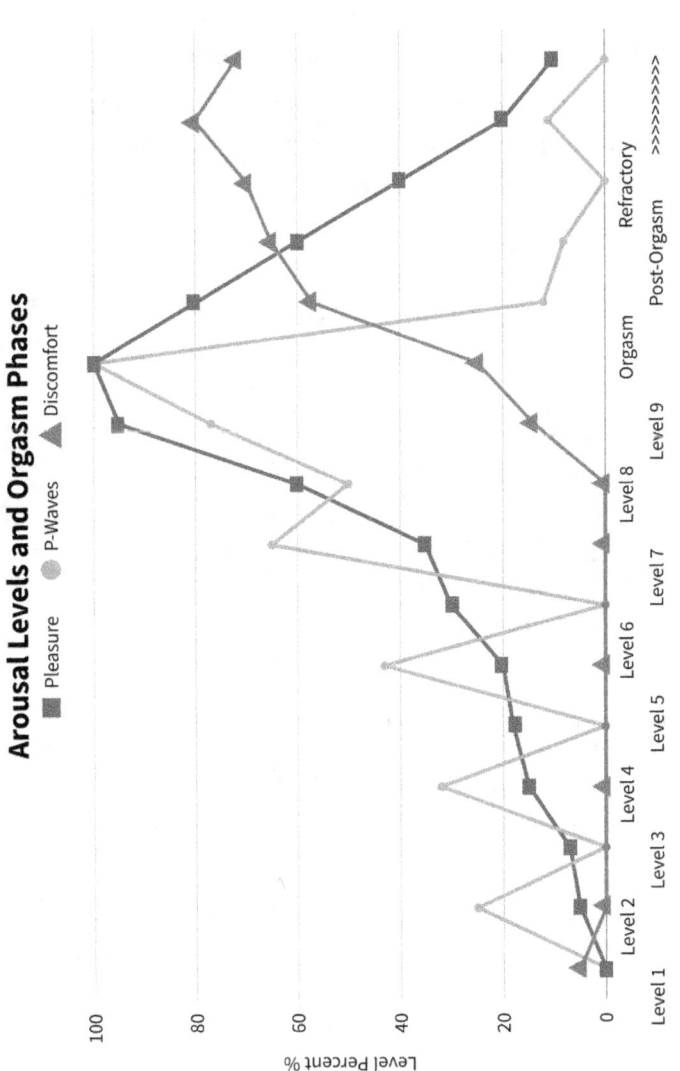

Understanding your levels of arousal throughout an orgasm cycle.

As you can see, the P-Waves rhythmically lead to orgasm. They still linger post-orgasm and into refractory. The pleasure rise is incremental, and the ridge of this line varies for everyone. Discomfort usually begins with insertion, but sometimes your hole will be so aroused and hungry, that you will not have any discomfort. For most, after a Super-O or wet orgasm, the discomfort grows. Again, everyone is wired differently.

Arousal Level	Phase	Type of Anal Sensations	Type of Penile Sensations
Level 1	No real arousal sensations	No sensations	Flaccid
Level 2–3	Some-what aroused	Your prostate awakens somewhat	Erection grows
Level 4	Aroused and just getting started. You begin your first thoughts, imagin-ing cumming	Your prostate becomes enlarged, and you start to feel pressure there with light tingly sensations forming	Erection near full growth, precum forms
Level 5–6	More than aroused	Some P-Waves start to build, very light anal contractions, nerves between prostate and penis start to lightly involuntarily contract	Fully erect, precum forms
Level 7–8	Really aroused	Light to moderate P-Waves, mild to light anal contractions, tingly and light pulsating penis sensations begin to form, involuntarily contractions	More precum forms, small contractions form
Level 9	Highly aroused, near wet/dry emission phase	Steady P-Waves, strong anal contractions, slight phantom feelings of peeing or cumming form with tingly and stronger, pulsating penis sensations, involuntarily contractions	Longer and shorter contractions simultaneously form, testicles and erection tighten

Level 9.5 – 9.9	"No turning back phase" — the instance you realize you are about to orgasm. Pre-orgasm contracting begins	Strong uncontrollable P-Waves, intense anal contractions, phantom feelings of peeing or cumming from, involuntarily contractions	Involuntary ejaculation spurts possible, short/intense contractions begin
Level 10	Full orgasm	P-Gasm (e.g., HFDO, HFWO, Super-O)	Ejaculation, heavy contracting

Remember, these results may not be the same for everyone. And not every session will be the same. Arousal levels depend on several factors, including an individual's mental state, hormone levels, and blood flow, etc. Some ride straight to Level 10, then drop to Level 8 before shooting up to Level 11. Others bounce from Level 10 down to Level 2, then back up to only Level 9. And some? They hit Level 10, pass out in the elevator, and their spouse comes home to find their feet stuck in the lobby doors.

Orgasm Styles

It can't be stated enough: **EVERYONE ORGASMS DIFFERENTLY**. The only thing that will be universal is the contracting of pelvic floor muscles. Some researchers have qualified them into three distinct types: wave orgasm, avalanche orgasm, or volcano orgasm.

The **wave** is consecutive contractions of tension and release at orgasm that lessen as you reach the refractory period. An **avalanche** occurs when the pelvic floor muscles have the highest tension, leading to a sudden dumping-like orgasm. A **volcano** orgasm releases when the pelvic floor muscles are at a lower tension before dramatically increasing and exploding as they tighten fully.

Did you know? Prostrate orgasms are very similar to women's G-Spot and clitoral orgasms. The prostate is similar to the urethral sponge material (G-Spot) of a biological women. And the frenulum (penis head) is similar to the clitoral cells and structure.

To follow are the most common types of stimulation to achieve orgasm:

1. **Tickling/tapping** (aka "guitar finger"): Using a finger (come hither technique) or toy, this style of orgasm is usually either a very rapid climax, or a slow build, fun climax.

2. **Thrusting:** Using fingers or a dildo will work. This method is usually the preferred method for anal enthusiasts. Some need deep penetration, others prefer short, shallow thrusts; or a varied combination of both.

3. **Vibrating:** With all the various toys available, revving up the motor on any vibrator to a high speed will get your prostate buzzing, and your cock spilling frothy milk.

4. **E-stim:** Experts in electrical pleasure-seeking use electrodes and a plug to send intense contractions to the prostate and cock at the same time. The feeling is blurred between pain and pleasure, and this orgasm is very addictive if you can master the right voltage and placement of electricity.

5. **Clenching/Mental:** For advanced users, this method

generally uses an Aneros (or no toy at all) and the mind to induce beautiful and surreal orgasms.

Remember, it all comes down to experimenting with the right anal physics and tuning into your body's natural responses. Personally, my primary method is thrusting. However, I still incorporate the others into my routine and even have created hybrid adaptations of these styles. I also enjoy starting with one method, then progressing to thrusting, i.e., start with clenching, then vibrating, then thrusting.

> For some cis gender women, anal sex applies perfect pressure to the anterior wall of the vagina (located right beneath the bladder). This deep pressure close to the cervix hits the anterior fornix. This is known as the "A-Spot" and it produces similar wave-like contractions. For all genders, drawn-out pushing in one place, versus continual thrusting can also help bring a more intense orgasm.

Whatever type you have, remember this: an orgasm is an orgasm is an orgasm, and so on. In short, **it does not matter how you arrive, or what vehicle gets you there, just learn how to drive and arrive at your orgasmic destination.**

CHAPTER 9

A TYPICAL SESSION

Overview

Your first raw, unfiltered look at what really happens behind closed doors—it's time to get meta and break the fourth wall!

I am often asked about my anal routine . . .

To get me in the right mood, I usually edge first, for 20-60 minutes. Other times I do nothing except wait a few days between ejaculating and anal play. If I abstain 10 days, I will usually go right into anal play with no masturbation.

Once in a while, I enjoy holding back from masturbation and anal play for 10 or more days. This heightened sensitivity propels me into Super-O nirvana, making the experience both deeply physical and intensely emotional. It often transforms a session into something that feels more like a spiritual, almost drug-induced journey.

In between abstaining and playing, I use an **Aneros** (or a similar type of toy). Sometimes I wear it at night and during sleep; sometimes I walk around the house or work on the computer. I will occasionally use it for an anal orgasm session; these sessions usually go for 1-2 hours and are more of an anal meditation and energy orgasm adventure. An alternative to my Aneros is the e-stim setup I use. I wrap the electrode pads around my penis, on the base of the perineum, and use an e-stim plug for my ass. This is super fun to use watching porn or just resting in bed. However, after about 20 minutes, it may start to feel uncomfortable and cause numbness.

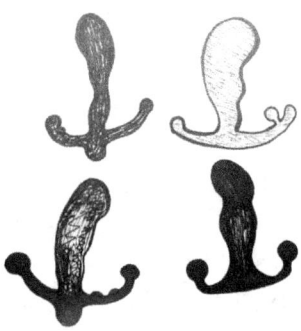

Aneros art. This is what they generally look like in real life, minus my hand-drawn embellishments.

As for my primary equipment and technique, it is all about automation for me. I prefer the dorsal recumbent position (back on the bed, knees bent at 35 degrees). Typically, I use a high-end **sex machine** and a curved silicone G-Spot/P-Spot dildo (flared at the base) with balls on the end to hit my perineum. This makes the sensations stronger. I might soak the dildo in hot water or put it in the microwave for a minute to get it warm. I use thick lube (silicone and water-based is my favorite), and slip it in. This is when I check in with myself to see how I feel mentally and physically. If everything is a go, I usually do a few deep breaths, maybe watch some "hands-free cumming" porn to get inspired, or go into my breathwork routines. Then I set the machine on the lowest level and add more lube.

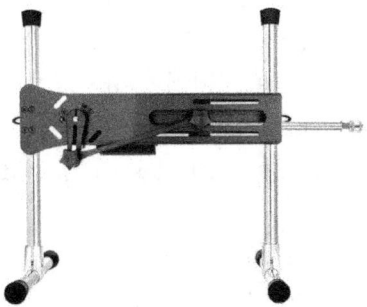

If there was a prostrainer army, the Hismith sex machine would be standard issued for battle.

The P-Waves immediately hit me, and an anal orgasm arrives within seconds. These dry anal orgasms build with more pleasure and intensity, increasing every five minutes. At this point, I close my eyes and my senses heighten. I usually precum instantly, and as I reach the 5-9 Arousal Levels, leaking occurs with occasional hard squirts of semen, prostatic fluid, and/or urine. As I build up my orgasms, I use my pelvic floor muscles to squeeze the liquids out of me. I use a combination of kegels and reverse kegels at varying levels and rates of frequency. I also ride the waves of each phase, pushing down on the dildo so the base hits my perineum, and I feel a full stretch of my hole. In addition, I move my hips up, lift my legs, squeeze them together; or widen them, to find the perfect spot to increase pressure on my prostate. I focus on my breath to slow it down as much as possible, and really relax my face, hands, legs and other muscles so I melt away into a trance. This combined effort usually sends me over the edge to reach orgasm.

Since the sweet spot of my prostate can move around, I am always adjusting the thrusts to find the best pleasure combinations; sometimes this involves making waves with my pelvic muscles and anal insertions. My Super-O, or final anal orgasm, occurs between 20-60 minutes of play. By then my prostate has become slightly sore, so I stop. Sometimes, after 10 minutes, I am able to start again. However, I usually find it difficult to have any more strong anal orgasms after a giant, long Super-O.

As mentioned, I've had sessions go for over 2 hours, but those are rare because of the soreness and discomfort from the dildo and thrusting. Depending on the session, I might engage in penile play and have a wet orgasm during or right after my Super-O. Sometimes I stop and feel so satisfied that I want to save my penile orgasm for my partner; or have it later in the day. It all depends on my mood, and what my body feels like it wants to do.

I also enjoy playing with my **percussion gun** attachment using a smaller P-Spot dildo (medium/firm silicone grade). I wrap it in a firm pillow (u-shaped), sit down on it, and ride away until the vibrations of my perineum, testes, prostate, and penis head can't take it anymore. I cum usually in minutes from this technique. It literally shakes the cum out of you! I call this "prostquaking".

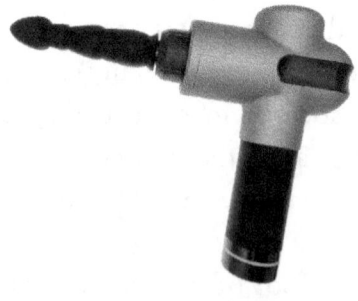

Percussion gun with attachment

The njoy Pure Wand is another great toy (*see section in TOYS for different ways to use it*) that I enjoy. I can go anywhere from 5-30 minutes with it. Sometimes I need a quick and easy P-Gasm and HFDO session, and this toy delivers. It is easy to set up and use.

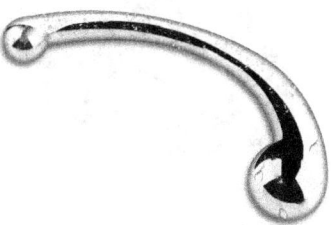

Curved prostate wand

The **Tremor** recently became part of my "tool shed". It is similar to a Sybian or MotorBunny straddle and ride machine. For the rideable attachments, I purchased the Motorbunny Premium Silicone Clit Stim XL Attachment; I also have the Bad Dragon, Flint® the Uncut Studded Dragon. Both are big and fill you up! I place the electric saddle on a wooden chest below the end of my bed (so it is almost 3 inches lower than the top of my mattress). Then I lie back on my bed, putting my knees on the edge of the wood chest so my legs are bent. The Tremor vibrates from a rocking motion, and it has a rolling setting as well that makes the attachment toy do circles. This sensation makes me cum hard when I am in the right state of mind.

But some days it doesn't work for me. Either way, I love it because it delivers a completely different prostate experience than my other toys. And when it does work for me, the orgasms come fast, hard and every 10-20 seconds. I can only do around 20-40 minutes with this setup.

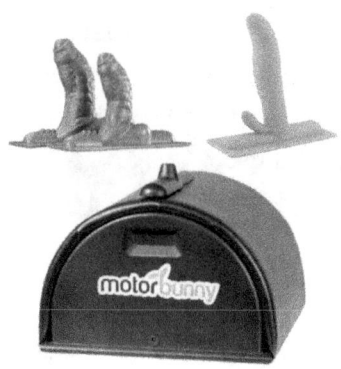

Motorbunny and Bad Dragon rideable attachments

Lastly, when the mood is right, I love getting into A-less and Mindgasm sessions with nipple play (*See the Mindgasm and A-Less section for details*). These are mental and almost spiritual orgasms. I put on my headphones and let my mind be the toy. Or I use sound arousal to let my imagination make me cum—I also love a good hypnosis file to guide me.

With any of the aforementioned methods, I am usually using my body to sync with the toy and waves of pleasure—I actively ride the toy during orgasms, creating centipede motions. And I breathe in a circular and deep pattern. I am always tuning in for loops and waves of pleasure, chasing them to a crescendo. Doing nipple play also helps to enhance the sessions. I see it as being a pilot at the controls, constantly adjusting and fine-tuning every detail.

Those are the methods that consistently deliver me bliss. But as the saying goes, "Your results may vary." Finding these reliable techniques was a process of trial and error, filled with surprises and lessons along the way. I wholeheartedly encourage you to build your own theme park of pleasure. Dive into the tricks I've shared—each holds the promise of unique sensations. Experiment with a diverse range of sex toys, each with its own mysteries and charm. Tailor-make your exploration, crafting a journey toward your ultimate adventure. This is not merely a recommendation; it's an invitation to a thrilling voyage of personal discovery and profound enjoyment. Each step forward is a step toward mastering your own orgasmic universe.

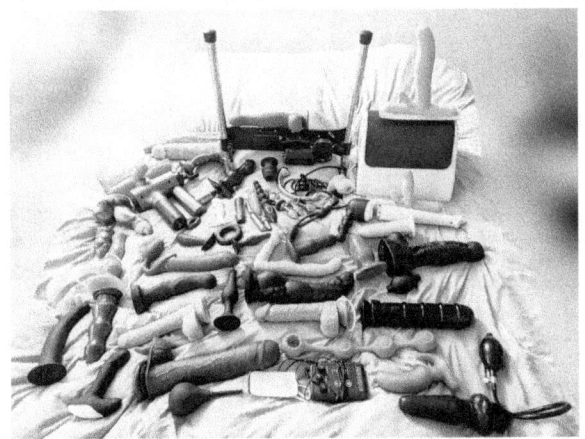

An assortment of WMD's (Weapons of Mass Delight)

PATH TO PROGRESSION FLOWCHART

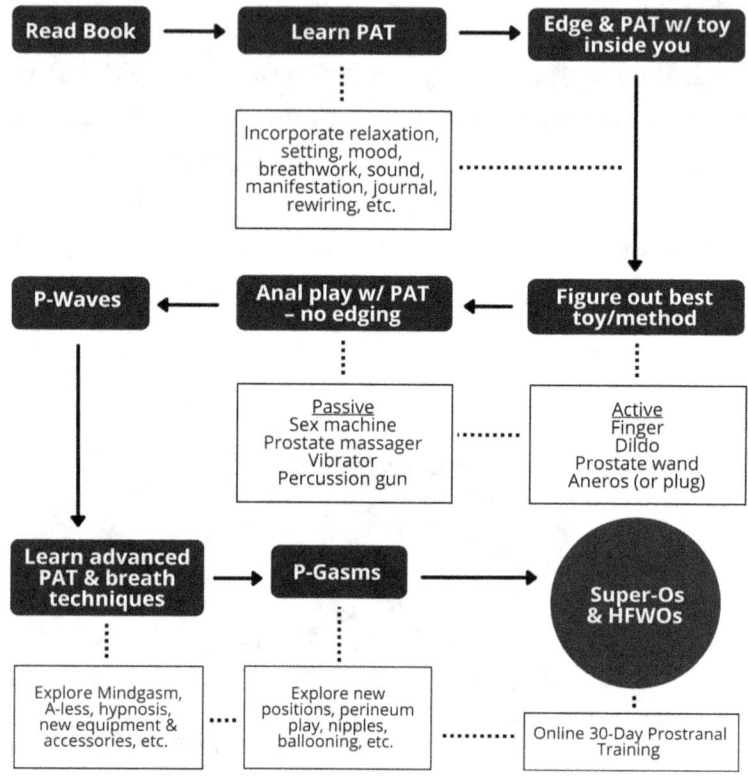

The flowchart provides a clear progression pathway. Reading the book takes an average of 5–11 hours (about 6–27 days). Start by mastering kegel exercises using the PAT Method. Setting the right environment for each session is also crucial. Practice edging by touching your penis while using a toy (like a plug or Aneros) and applying PAT techniques at high arousal levels. Squeeze and clench, imagining reaching orgasm through kegels. Once comfortable, explore the right toy or method—this could be your finger or a sex machine. A passive approach is recommended so you can relax and focus on subtle sensations. At this stage, stop touching yourself and focus on anal play with PAT techniques until you start feeling P-Waves. As P-Waves become more consistent and easier to trigger, use advanced PAT practice and breathwork techniques. You can also incorporate A-less exercises from Chapter 20. Over time, you'll experience various P-Gasms. In parallel, explore Mindgasm techniques, hypnosis, new positions, and perineum stimulation. This all leads to Super-Os and HFWOs. The 30-Day Prostranal Training is also a great way to get there quicker. Consistent practice at each stage is the key to mastery.

CHAPTER 10

MASSAGE SERVICES

Overview

- Understand the different types of massages and what to expect.
- Learn about focused prostate massage and its benefits.
- Prepare to realize you've been living under a rock and that you haven't traveled enough.

Did you know that therapeutic prostate massage has been performed for thousands of years around the world—particularly in Asia? In fact, prostate play originated with royalty. Every king, shah, and sultan with a harem typically had a monk or private doctor perform prostate massages—much like a sex coach/guru. The purpose was to turn the royal man into a well-conditioned and excellent lover.

Today, anyone can experience this pleasure, with many massage options available. Let's explore the differences between therapeutic, sensual, and erotic sessions.

Every state and country are different—research the laws in your area before you go seek out any massage service!

A **therapeutic massage** session focuses on physical well-being, muscle tension relief, and overall relaxation. It is often performed by licensed professionals trained in various techniques like Swedish, deep tissue, or myofascial release. The goal is to improve circulation, reduce pain, and enhance mobility. If prostate massage is incorporated in a therapeutic setting, it is typically done for medical reasons, such as improving prostate health, relieving pelvic tension, or assisting with chronic conditions like prostatitis. There is no sexual intent in therapeutic sessions, and boundaries are strictly professional.

A **sensual massage** blends relaxation with heightened body awareness and gentle arousal. It focuses on pleasure, touch sensitivity, and energy flow, rather than direct sexual stimulation. Sensual massages often involve slow, intentional strokes, body-to-body contact, and deep relaxation techniques. In the context of prostate massage, the goal may be to help the receiver become more comfortable with new sensations, encourage arousal without pressure, and allow for deeper connection with one's body. Some tantric practitioners incorporate sensual elements to enhance pleasure, but climax is not the main focus—instead, it's about building arousal and expanding pleasure over time.

An **erotic massage** is explicitly focused on sexual pleasure and arousal. This type of session may include direct genital stimulation, prostate play, and orgasmic release. The intent is to heighten pleasure, explore erogenous zones, and sometimes introduce new experiences, such as full-body orgasms, prostate orgasms, or tantric energy releases. Erotic massages are usually provided in private settings, and while some professionals offer them discreetly, they are often considered outside the realm of regulated massage therapy. It's important to research providers carefully, establish clear boundaries, and ensure mutual consent to create a safe and satisfying experience.

A professional sensual or erotic masseuse will most likely provide tantric Lingham and prostate massage. Beyond style and training, these sessions differ in intent, techniques, and boundaries. An experienced masseuse can teach you many things about your prostate and help awaken it. Best of all, a good prostate massage **facilitates sexual health, improving circulation, and promoting detoxification by stimulation of the genital areas and prostate**. It cultivates breath awareness, enhances receptivity, and connects with erogenous zones around the pelvic floor, extending outward to relax both body and mind. Just sit back, let go, and fully immerse yourself in the pleasure.

Typically, these massages last around 60 minutes, and the practitioner will dedicate the last 20 minutes to your prostate. It often includes external massaging of the perineum and anus with warm oil in a circular motion using gentle pressure. This includes gentle rubbing, teasing, and scratching with the fingertips. These varied techniques are performed throughout your prostate massage for maximum pleasure. Once properly relaxed and stimulated, a gloved finger is gently inserted into the anus to gently rub the rectum wall and stroke the prostate. Slowly, the tip of the finger gets inserted several times in a teasing manner to help you relax and grow accustomed to the feeling. As you relax and become more aroused, deeper exploration naturally follows until the prostate and seminal vesicles are reached, allowing for gentle massage and milking. With time, your masseuse will learn about your body and help you achieve various types of prostate orgasms; they can even incorporate prostate toys in their sessions.

Knowing what you want from a session—whether it's relaxation, heightened sensitivity, or orgasmic release—will help you communicate better with your masseuse. Find a practitioner aligned with your intentions. I recommend seeking a Tantra-trained Dakini for best results. They act as a guide, healer, and teacher who helps people deepen their connection to pleasure, self-awareness, and spiritual growth.

If this topic gets you excited, I recommend visiting **eroticmassage.com**. This educational platform focuses on teaching erotic massage and sensual touch techniques. It offers over 20 hours of instructional videos, featuring demonstrations by professionals. The content includes courses such as "Anal Massage" and specialized techniques like "Mapping: Practicing Placement of Attention," which emphasizes applying finger pressure in a focused, structured way to specific points on the body for somatic (body sensation) awareness. The site caters to a wide audience, including lovers and professionals like Sexological Bodyworkers, with training materials used by practitioners.

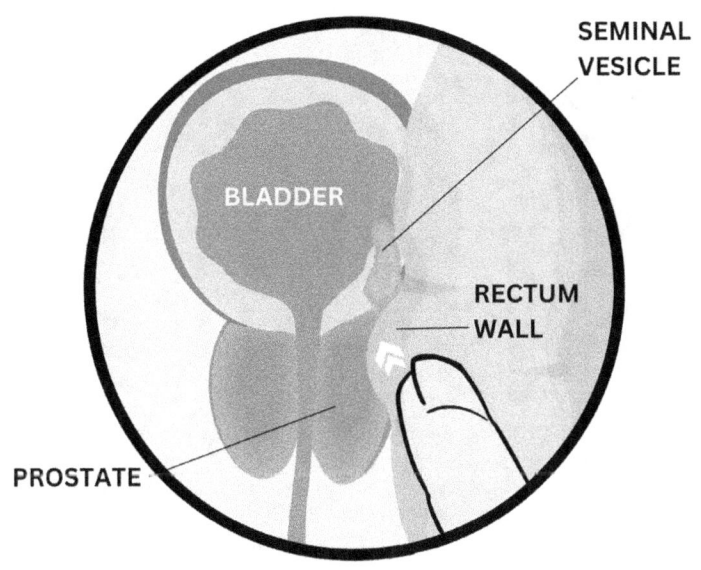

Massage here for best results.

CHAPTER 11

A GUIDE TO STRETCHING OUT

Overview

- Master stretching techniques for smooth, next-level progress.
- Pain is a signal to stop and you should listen to your body.
- Prioritize safety to have a comfortable and enjoyable experience.
- Realize that anal is basically giving birth in reverse—on repeat.

It takes time and practice to open up your anus. And much like a flower, you will need to be delicate when you begin stretching your "petals". Some of us are just tighter than others. Attempting to penetrate your ass with a large toy right away results in a painful and less-than-positive experience. So, start small! And always moisturize in between sessions (*see "Lube, Aftercare" section*).

Many people believe they are too tight to enjoy anal sex. This is not true. For both men and women, many of us have been conditioned from an early age to believe that our "dirty backdoor" is off-limits for any kind of insertion.

With that said, a butt plug and lots of lube is the perfect place to start when learning to stretch your hole. Once the plug slips past the widest section, the initial discomfort should subside, and you can start to enjoy that inexpressible feeling of fullness. After slowly plunging it in and out a few times, make sure to begin your PAT (kegel) exercises. As you kegel, search for sensations of pleasure around pelvic area, anus, genitalia, and other parts of your body. Leaving the plug in for as long as comfortable (20 minutes, 2 hours, or all day) will help with a moderate and consistent stretching effect. It is best to buy a training kit (available at a sex toy store online, or a local store) so you can graduate as you become more comfortable with increasingly larger-sized plugs.

Or, try a set of dilators; and start with the smallest size first. Dilators with graduated sizes will help you with your backdoor training sessions. They come in all shapes and sizes e.g., tapered, plugged, etc. This training regimen will help you gradually build up your tolerance so you can take different-sized toys. Remember to take your time and stretch daily. You will be surprised at how quickly you can handle other sizes. I highly recommend the b-Vibe Snug Plug toys (sizes 1-6) for your first dilator kit. They are perfect to use as butt plugs as well.

> Anal plugs are the multi-tool for prostrainers. Depending on the type of plug, they can provide prostate stimulation while walking around, give the feeling of being full, or even just to train and stretch that hole. You might

even enjoy the naughty feeling of walking around in public. Some plugs give prostate stimulation, and others just stretch. But feeling full can be enjoyable whenever you want to engage your anal nerve endings.

When you are ready to buy your first dildo, start with something about the size of the midpoint of your butt plug diameter. You do not want it to be too big. Just like going to the gym, never grab the heaviest weight and start lifting. The circumference of your first dildo might be slightly uncomfortable when first inserting it, but once you relax and go slowly, the initial discomfort will subside. Always use lots of lube and practice with the dildo 3-4 times per week for around 10 to 30 minutes. **You will be surprised how quickly your anus will adapt to it.** In time, you will look forward to your stretching sessions, and you should start getting steady flows of precum.

After a few weeks, you could buy something a little bigger. Or try one with different curves, shapes, and ridges, etc. Feel free to keep expanding your comfort zone with regular practice. Depending on your practice schedule and your ability to relax, each dildo may take a few weeks to get accustomed to during anal play. Scale up in size little by little, until you find the feeling of fullness that best fits you. Personally, anything larger than 2.25 inches in diameter (7 inches in circumference) is challenging. But everyone is different, so experiment and find your limits. And remember that there is no need to go bigger. It is totally up to you what goes up you. But if you do resize your dildo, do it accordingly. I highly recommend buying a stretching dildo that tapers, like an inner band trainer, or a large cone to learn your comfort level.

Recommended 10-Day Anal Dilation Schedule

Day	Toy/ Dilator Size	Duration (Minutes)	Notes
1	Smallest	5–10	Focus on relaxation, deep breathing, and inserting just the tip.
2	Smallest	10	Insert slightly deeper, pause if tense, and hold until relaxed.
3	Smallest	10–15	Aim for full insertion, move slowly, and rest if needed.
4	Smallest	15	Maintain full insertion, practice gentle in-and-out motion.
5	Next Size Up	5–10	Insert just the tip. Focus on adjusting to the new size.
6	Next Size Up	10	Gradually increase depth, stop if resistance is too strong.
7	Next Size Up	10–15	Work toward full insertion, relax pelvic muscles throughout.
8	Next Size Up	15	Hold comfortably, practice slight movement to build tolerance.
9	Next Size Up	15	Assess comfort—stay at this size if needed before progressing again.
10	Evaluate	10–15	Either maintain size or move to the next size if ready. Decide if bigger is better for pleasure or if it diminishes pleasure. Repeat 10-day schedule for medium or larger toys if you choose to go bigger.

Only increase size when the current one feels comfortable and manageable. If soreness occurs, take a break and resume when ready — don't force it and go slow. It could take more than 10 days for some to level up. I recommend a dilator kit with either 5-8 dilators if you want to go slower and are tighter

The anus is naturally elastic, designed to

stretch for pooping (up to 2 inches in diameter). It can, however, expand significantly past this threshold and be stretched up to 4-5 inches in diameter with training. The Guinness World Record for the largest anal stretch is set at 9.5 inches in diameter. Attempting such dangerous stretching carries serious risks, including muscle damage and loss of function. Do **not** try this!

Stretch your hole with a smaller object beforehand until you can fit the dildo. Use a preferred position or method that helps you take it in more easily and go slow. **CAUTION: Never put anything inside of you where you risk ripping your anus!** Once you tear the anal area, it can take months to heal. Speak to a doctor about safely stretching and stimulating your ass. Ultimately, anal stretching is about training your pelvic floor and abdomen to relax. You need to train your nerves and body to get past the panic point and stay fully relaxed during penetration. And always follow the Golden Rule of prostate play: **Never continue when you feel pain!**

As you become more comfortable, you will find what type of stretch feels best for your choice of toy. I found there are two types of happiness in your hole:

A) The feeling of fullness; or

B) The feeling of space and movement.

For some, it can be both. Or it can depend on your mood. The joyful feeling of fullness happens when your toy (usually a larger one) makes your hole feel so tight that there is barely any room for lube. It makes your prostate, bladder, rectum, ejaculatory duct, and seminal vesicles feel like they are packed on a subway at rush hour with the hottest models surrounding you. Every push and pull brings near-aching but delicious pleasure. It creates the perfect border between pain and ecstasy.

> Before you know it, the idea of putting a toy inside you will become completely exhilarating. And when it enters, there will be no pain. You will feel full and happy.

On the other hand, the feeling of space and movement, occurs when the toy has room to move around your anal cavity. It allows you to "bite down" on it for extra sensation, or just let it ride and skip along the grove of your prostate.

In terms of stamina, the size of the toy directly correlates with the level of stretching, providing greater potential for fatigue due to clenching. Stamina and receptiveness depend on your ability to encourage your anus to remain flexible. This principle also applies to sensitivity. By focusing on the essence of your pleasure while maintaining awareness of bodily tension, you can explore the realm of non-clenching anal pleasure.

But be warned! You could lose that stretch over time. If you go larger and stop, don't expect to get back into ramming those larger toys back in right away. Even if you take only a few weeks away from your regular toy, it will feel snug again and might even hurt. **The moral of the story is: Always go slow and never stick things in quickly.** You'll become an "anal virgin" again faster than you realize, especially when you stop stretching your hole.

Worst of all, repeated overstretching can weaken the anal sphincter, leading to difficulty controlling bowel movements and rectal prolapse (where part of the rectum slips out of place).

> The body naturally reacts by tightening up the pelvic floor and stopping something from entering your anus. You must teach your body to relax, controlling the reflex. This gets easier as you practice stretching your hole.

Some newcomers have shared that using anorectal products (containing less than 5% lidocaine) helped ease discomfort during their first experiences with penetration. These ointments typically combine a local anesthetic with a pain reliever or anti-inflammatory agent to reduce pain and irritation. However, **I strongly advise against this practice,** as it poses a significant risk of injury. Numbing lubricants can desensitize the area excessively, not only increasing the chance of harm but also diminishing pleasure by blocking sensation entirely.

Size and Depth Training

Remember that some anal discomfort can be expected as you are learning. Pain, however, is not a pathway to pleasure. Always listen to your body! Some new prostrainers have gotten hurt early on—similar to a newbie in the gym's weight room going all-out the first week. **Tearing your ass (aka anal fissure) can lead to serious issues** and keep you on the sidelines for a long time. Be very careful if you decide to push the limits of size and depth with your toys.

Some consider this field to be a form of body modification. You need to know that it comes with risks of physical damage that can even be permanent. I strongly suggest moderation in everything you try. *Anal* and *pain* and are two words that should never go together!

Common tools I do not recommend for this type of play are:

- **Inflatables** — Pumping up your toy can be fun and intriguing. Since they size up with each pump, there is no need to buy several different-sized dildos. **BUT BEWARE: they are very dangerous because you can over-inflate and blow out your ass like a bike tire!** Therefore, I highly-recommend avoiding inflatable toys.

- **Colon Snakes** — These long, flexible anal toys can be 3-5 feet long and are much thinner than regular dildos. They are soft and tapered, and they easily bend to follow your body's natural internal curves. As with most toys, there are varying types available. Colon Snakes can cause serious internal damage. Again, I suggest avoiding them since they are very dangerous and do not stimulate the prostate.

- **Fists and XXL Dildos** — Obviously, the range of dildos available can satisfy prostainers looking for XXL adventures. There is no shortage or limit here. Fisting usually requires another person and brings with it a world of dangers. Not only can fists tear your anus, but you have to worry about sharp fingernails and trusting another person to not damage you. That is why I also do not encourage large dildo play and fisting as kinks.

The value of prostate pleasure is not there, and the risk of injury is high.

To wrap up this section on different training tools and methods, I wanted to make sure you've got all the right information on this subject. There are a few other tools I didn't cover because, frankly, they pose a high risk of injury. **I'm all about keeping things safe and sound. I suggest avoiding depth training and sticking to the things I've covered that provide safe, direct anal stimulation.**

Here is a quick recap . . .

Safe Ways to Stimulate & Stretch	Avoid Doing This
Start small, slowly and lots of lube	Pushing into your pain boundaries
Stretch daily and not when you are sore	Using anorectal products containing lidocaine
Use dilators or band trainers if you want to go bigger	Shoving it in quickly with not enough lube
Find your favorite feeling (fullness or space)	Playing with inflatables, colon snakes, fisting, XXL dildos, etc.

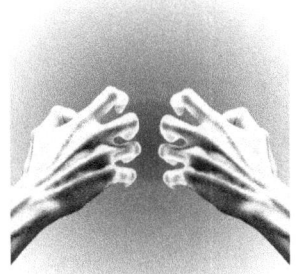

Goatse, the infamous 90's internet photo of a man stretching his anus to the diameter of a softball, probably took prostranal too far. Please never go full Goatse.

CHAPTER 12

FINDING YOUR PROSTATE & THE TYPES OF PROSTATE

Overview

- Learn to locate your prostate and how its unique sensations enhance pleasure.
- Enjoy my poetic take on prostates and the rectum—like a wine snob raving about notes of cherry and tobacco.

As men get older, the prostate increases in size. Younger men generally have smaller ones, and it might be more difficult to find the prostate without arousal. Regardless, different prostates react differently to stimulation.

Using your finger, go inside and figure out where it is. Or, have a partner help you explore. **Once you understand the topography and type of prostate, you will better know what type of toy and stimulation works best to find your "magic button".** This will help when you start exploring with your toys.

The prostate is not located in the anus; rather, it sits just below the bladder, in front of the rectum, and surrounds the urethra. While the prostate itself is not within the anus, access to it is possible through the rectum, which provides a pathway for examination or stimulation. To clarify, you can't touch it directly. The prostate organ is safely located behind the rectal wall, meaning it can be accessed indirectly by applying pressure through the rectum.

To perform a basic prostate massage, gently insert a finger or toy into the rectum, angling it slightly forward to apply gentle pressure to the general area where the prostate is located. Use a repeated in-and-out motion. Don't be discouraged if you don't feel anything significant right away. The prostate sits close to the bladder, so if you sense a slight urge to pee, you are likely in the right area.

Choosing the right tool is important for stimulation. You'll need something that can indirectly apply pressure to the prostate, with a firmer touch being more effective. It is essential to press firmly against the rectal wall to engage the prostate. Guide the finger or toy you're using toward the front of your groin area (toward the base of your penis), as the prostate is relatively shallow, about one to three inches inside, depending on your body. **Experiment with angles to find the most effective way to target your prostate.** Keep in mind that locating the prostate and getting pleasure from it are two separate experiences.

> **Pro Tip**: If you still struggle to find your prostate, try masturbating to ejaculate with your finger inside your ass. As you are cumming, feel around and your prostate should swell and be hard, even pulsating. Notice the

depth of your finger and remember where your prostate resides. Close your eyes to really tune in to the location so you can mark it on your imaginary map.

To better understand your own topography, here are some of the prostate types that I've taken the liberty to name:

"Contact Lens": Spongy, soft, and almost unnoticeable. Feels like it is surrounded by gelatin blobs that are trying to keep you from finding it. Mid length, around 2 inch inside. Very hard to locate.

"Pearl Ribbon": Runs deep along the anus and is very firm. Not easy to find due to its thin shape. Lightly ribbed, bumpy and almost off-center a bit. Shallow from entrance about 1 inch inside.

"Almond Jellyfish": Soft, smooth, and long ridge that widens and forms a coarse texture midway through. Close to the sphincter around 1 inch or so, almond-like in shape. Wet and spongy. Easy to find.

"Silk Rail": Close to the entrance of the rectum and super soft. Very easy to find and produces instant sensation when touched. Small and like a silky rail of ribbon. Medium density in feel, less than 1 inch inside the cavity.

"Triangle Pillow": Smooth feeling to it, deep to about 3 inches inside, yet accessible with a finger. There is a channel on one side, unequal-shaped. Challenging to find, a poofy and rounded-triangular shape.

"Toothpick": Deep and tricky to find, and almost camouflages with the cavity. Sandpaper feel. A flat, thin ridge that is very deep, anywhere from 1-3 inches inside.

"Inverted Walnut": Shallow, but difficult to get to without hooking a finger. Feels squishy but becomes erect quickly. Likes pressure to roll off the sides rather than rubbed directly on top of it. Goes long and deep into the cavity.

"Curveball": Deep and soft with some bumps like seams. Smooths out deeper down but also curves up. Easy to find, but it moves when you play with it and becomes evasive. Goes in about 1-2 inches inside.

Exploring the prostate reveals a world as fascinating as human fingerprints. Each one has its own structure and sensations. It helps you see what we all have in common while appreciating our unique differences. Learning about your prostate boosts your self-awareness and opens the door to a richer experience of pleasure. As you uncover more secrets about this small yet powerful gland, remember that knowing your body is the key to unlocking its full potential. So, approach this journey with curiosity, respect, and a sense of adventure—it's an exploration of one of the body's most underrated and remarkable wonders.

PROSTATE GALLERY

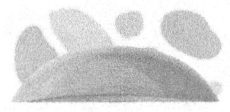

CONTACT LENS

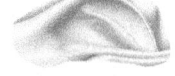

SILK RAIL

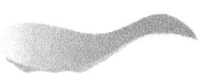

CURVEBALL

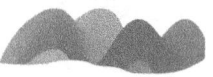

PEARL RIBBON

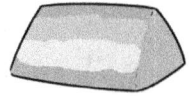

TRIANGLE PILLOW

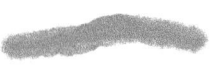

TOOTHPICK

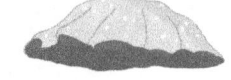

ALMOND JELLYFISH

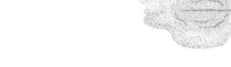

INVERTED WALNUT

CHAPTER 13

PREPARATION AND CLEANING

Overview

- Proper techniques for a safe and comfortable experience.
- Health and diet tips to support better preparation.
- Like the fossil fuel industry, there's an upstream and downstream—expect some mess when you hit the refinery.

Anal play requires some basic skills that are essential to learn. Similar to anal sex with a partner, you need to take a few precautions before the fun gets started. Here are the basics:

- Pee beforehand to empty the bladder as much as possible.
- Don't eat a giant carne asada burrito before your start your session!
- Buy some absorbent pads and have a towel to place under you during your sessions.

- Keep a roll of toilet paper handy in case of a fecal "surprise".
- Sanitize/wash your preferred toy before and after use.
- Have your lube ready and close by.

Some of the following sections, however, are more complicated and will take time to master.

> There is a saying: "You don't have anal sex with an ass full of shit for the same reason that you don't have oral sex with a mouth full of food."

Best Cleaning Methods

You will need to choose your method of cleaning your rectum:

- **Bidet/Shower Hose:** Hook this up to your toilet and use the spray handle to shoot water into your hole and clean it. This is a wise investment for your bathroom. Very practical and efficient. You can purchase them online for under $30 (USD).
- **Douche/Enema Bulbs:** Easy to store and nice for travel. Cheap, but not efficient.
- **Enema Bag:** These IV looking contraptions are slow and not fun to use, but they work. And some prostrainers love adding coffee for an extra cleansing feeling.
- **Plastic Bottle:** One day you will be somewhere and have nothing to clean your ass with. You will thank

me for this trick . . . it's not pretty and is hard to do, but it works. Take a full bottle of water and try to aim it up with one lucky squeeze. **Do not shove it inside and be very careful not to cut your rim!**

The bidet/shower hose is the best option. Count anywhere from 3-5 seconds when filling your hole with water, then gently squeeze it all out of your ass. Do not overfill past this count, or you'll get into the sigmoid colon and beyond. If you recall from a previous chapter's diagram, the sigmoid colon is the S-shaped section of the large intestine, right before the rectum. It's like a twisty storage tube that holds waste, helping compact it before you let it go. Think of it as the final curve in your gut's cleanup crew. If you get water past this area, you'll have a shit river to deal with and will need to do a full cleaning instead. Interaction with the sigmoid might also cause your intestines to unleash a slow, endless release of mud that prevents anal play for hours. **Avoid the sigmoid!**

If you plan for a quick anal session, then clean for around 10-25 minutes. If you feel your stomach is full and you plan on playing with your larger toys, aim for a full 30-minute cleanse. Either way, repeat until the water that comes out is clear. If it smells and/or there is any brown or yellow colored water when you squeeze the last drops out, there is still more shit inside your rectum.

You will need to squat, maybe even stand up to get all the water out.

If you did it correctly, it should sound like a flappy series of wet farts after each rinse. Put a small or medium-sized toy in afterward, standing over the toilet, and thrust several times to make sure that you were successful. This is like checking the oil in a car. You want no shit on your dildo. And even if you do all of what I've suggested, be aware that there can still be a surprise release of your bowels when you are 10 minutes into toying your ass.

Don't be scared of poop. It is natural and something you will need to overcome. You could see mucosa in the clean water (e.g., small traces of intestinal lining that look slimy and sticky). This is normal. **Blood, on the other hand, is no good!** See a doctor at once and stop what are you doing until you can determine the health issue.

Never rush the cleaning process. A good cleaning relaxes your anal muscles and gets them comfortable with the feeling of being penetrated before you start your prostate play sessions.

> Some "cheat" to avoid shitting themselves during play. They use psyllium husk powder mixed with water or anti-diarrheal medi- cine beforehand. This comes with its own risks and doesn't always work. I do **not** rec- ommend this!

Fiber is good for your diet. However, too much fiber can dehydrate you and cause cramps and/or hemorrhoids. Never take more than the recommended dose of fiber. **Make sure you drink plenty of water to stay hydrated all day long.** If you do this, your stools will be compact, making cleaning considerably easier, and you will spend less time over the toilet.

Loose and runny stools are difficult to clean out, no matter how much you clean up before anal play. And you might just have one of those days where you cannot completely clean yourself out. Eventually, you will discover the frustrating reality of your intestines and ass. Whenever you think you are clean, suddenly the second anal chamber opens and you have to douche again. **Some days it feels like you are fighting a river of endless sludge.**

The most frustrating experience is when you are mid-session in anal play and poop comes out after all the careful cleaning. You go back to the shower hose and try douching with water, then safely shove a lubed toy in your ass again to see if you got it all out this time, and return to play. But then it happens again: shit everywhere! I just quit on those days and laugh it off.

A final note on cleaning: **Do not forget to clean out your ass** after **play!** This can prevent bacteria, yeast, and other nasty things from forming. Use your method of cleaning, or even just a finger during your shower to get some water (no soap!) in there and wash out the lube.

THE ILLUSION ...

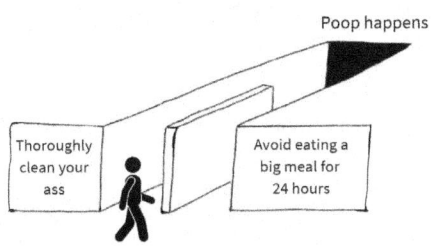

Poop happens

Thoroughly clean your ass

Avoid eating a big meal for 24 hours

EVERYTHING WILL BE FINE

Never start your anal sessions without some tissues or paper towels. Using puppy (incontinence) pads is also advised. No matter how much you prep, sometimes an unexpected event can occur.

CHAPTER 14

LUBE, LUBE, LUBE

Overview

- Proper lube techniques for a safe and comfortable experience.
- A breakdown of all the types available.
- Health and diet tips to support better preparation.
- Side note: The Summer Olympics could have a 50-meter swimming race in a pool full of lube to boost viewership.

Surprisingly, the anus has mucus glands that can help lubricate your ass. This is a natural process to help move excretion through your system. Anal play can activate these glands and make you "wet". Unfortunately for most, you cannot rely on it as a substitute for lube during anal play—you still need lube and lots of it. And **you can never have enough lube!** It is the currency of prostate play.

Types and Recommendations

Generally speaking, there are three types of lubrication:

- Water-based
- Silicone-based
- Oil-based

Find a water-based lube that is viscous. You want it thick, but not sticky—and you want it slippery, but not too watery. Stay away from silicone-based lube unless your toy allows it. Most silicone toys are not compatible with silicone lubes, which can ruin them. Many reports indicate that silicone lubricants can deteriorate soft, silicone sex toys due to the way that some silicone molecules react with other silicone materials. Personally, I've found that silicone tends to get on your sheets and clothing, which leaves them ruined (except for the hybrid silicone/water-based ones). The only good thing about silicone is that you rarely have to reapply after initial use. The other downside is that it gets all over the shower when you rinse off and can create a slipping hazard.

If you choose to go with water-based lubes, you might want to buy a lube injector. Use the blue plastic model syringe to avoid having to reapply lube every 2-5 minutes. Shooting a healthy dose of lube before anal helps keep things juicy for a long time.

The other alternative is oil-based lubes. Some love olive, coconut, vegetable cooking oil, Shea butter, etc. Oil-based lubes are much less expensive and easy to locate and purchase. While these derived oils can feel great, some of the synthetic ingredients such as petroleum or mineral oils can cause skin irritations. Some people have serious glycerin allergies, so read the labels carefully. I recommend against them as they are harder to wash off, potentially leading to bacterial infections.

And then there are the homemade mixes . . .

The most popular lube among die-hard anal prostrainers is J-Lube. Get J-Lube (the powdered stuff) and make your own if you are a DIY type. It is cheap and, again, you can never have enough lube. It can make gallons of lube. J-Lube is excellent because you can mix it to different consistencies. However, preparing the right consistency can be difficult for first-time users; so check online for good homemade recipes and instructions. J-Lube is typically used by farmers and veterinarians, as well as for special effects artists. Many love it because it sticks to the skin well (i.e., extremely slippery) and you don't need much.

As for safety, J-Lube is comprised of sucrose and polyethylene oxide (known as PEG-90M, it is used as a thickener for lotions, shampoos, cosmetics, etc.). It is considered to have low toxicity and to be non-irritating. But some say you should be careful if you are a diabetic, prone to yeast infections, scared of possible PEG-90M exposure, etc. Conduct further research if you are concerned. I recommend against J-Lube since it is not FDA approved for humans.

The FDA (Food and Drug Administration) regulates personal lubricants as Class II medical devices. This means lubes must meet specific safety standards, including biocompatibility testing, condom compatibility, and microbiological safety assessments before they can be sold. Always check for FDA clearance, often listed as "510(k) approved", on the label.

A mixture of J-Lube and Crisco, or coconut oil, is also something prostrainers use for heavy-duty anal play. They work as differentials and slide against each other nicely. They're sometimes used by those who enjoy fisting, since the oil seals the forearm and slips against the J-Lube. (But like I said earlier, fisting is dangerous. I do not recommend it or this lube mixture.)

There are prostrainers who enjoy using cornstarch lube. It is easy to make and fun to use. Some will say that cornstarch can lead to a yeast infection. But most studies have disproved this and found that cornstarch prevents your body from having an environment conducive to an apathogenic yeast. If you feel like being a scientist, go ahead and make a batch.

You will need the following ingredients:

- 2-4 teaspoons of cornstarch—add more cornstarch if you want a stickier lube, but the minimum should be two teaspoons
- 1 cup of water
- A container to boil it in (e.g., a pan or a pot)
- A plastic container to store the lube once it cools

The process takes only 10 to 20 minutes. Just mix the cornstarch and one cup of water in the pan or pot. Use two teaspoons of cornstarch to start. Add more teaspoons if the mixture looks too transparent or light for you. Continuously stir the mixture until the pot or pan is boiling. This is important since there will be lumps if the mixture is not constantly stirred. No one wants lumpy lube! Let it cool but do not place it inside a refrigerator or freezer since this affects the consistency and will create lumping. After it cools, pour it into a plastic container. (Again, I do not recommend using this lube but if you want to do a quick science experiment, have fun!)

While we are at it, let's talk about fake cum lube (external only). Here's a simple, quick recipe for fake semen using common kitchen ingredients:

- 1 cup of water
- 1 tablespoon of cornstarch
- Pinch of baking powder and J-Lube
- A pinch of salt (optional, for added realism)

The instructions are simple:

- In a small saucepan, mix the water and cornstarch, J-Lube, and baking powder until fully dissolved.
- Heat the mixture over low to medium heat, stirring continuously to avoid lumps.
- Remove from heat and let it cool. If it's too thick, add a bit of water to thin it out. If it's too thin, reheat and add a little more cornstarch.

(Safety Note: This mixture is safe for external use but should not be ingested or used internally as it is not sterilized. Always ensure the mixture is cooled completely before use.)

Lastly, let's talk about numbing creams. Many numbing lubes can also be used as a lube. They contain a chemical numbing agent designed to desensitize the anal wall, creating less pain and discomfort. The added ingredient is typically benzocaine; a topical agent that temporarily blocks nerve signal pain. Numbing creams do not always have the same effect on everyone, and some of the additional chemicals in those formulas can be unsafe. The downside is the loss of sensation during the riding part, which takes away pleasure. Some believe it could be a good way to "break the virginity seal" for the first few sessions. If you choose to use a numbing cream, use only FDA approved ones and talk with a doctor. I still advise against numbing creams.

Lube Technique

A lube syringe or "lube launcher" is a recommended purchase. This slim injector makes it super easy and comfy to prepare for anal play. Just stick the tip into your favorite lube and pull back the plunger to fill up the syringe. Once it's loaded, insert the "needle" into the spot you want to lube, then push the plunger to release the lubrication. Simple as that!

Method #1: After cleaning your rectum, inject a moderate amount of lube in your hole, as deep as your injector lets you. Form a pocket of lube inside your rectum, but not too much that it is uncomfortable. For me, I do 2 to 3 pumps. Have the lube sit for a while. Feel your body for signals of a bowel movement. If so, use the toilet and push it out. Sometimes you get a lube with feces, sometimes a few mucous trails, or sometimes you get only lube. This helps lubricate your inner walls, making shit less likely to stick instead of coming out. Make sure to re-inject lube afterwards and get back into action when you feel it is time.

Method #2: If you choose not to use a lube injector, then keep a full bottle with a pump near your play area. You will often need to reapply lube every 2-5 minutes depending on your setup and the toy's material. After a while, you will need less and less. I can never say enough that you can never use enough lube. So do not be conservative when reapplying.

Aftercare Lubrication

Once the toys and lube are put away, proper aftercare is key to staying healthy. Anal marathons can leave you feeling raw. Take time to care for your body to prevent irritation and promote healing for future sessions. Gently clean the outside of your anal area with warm water and a mild, fragrance-free soap. Avoid harsh scrubbing, as the delicate skin around it can be sensitive. Keep your body hydrated to help with tissue recovery. Drink plenty of water and leave your ass alone for at least 24 hours. For those seeking additional relief, Dr. Tush's Signature After Butt Play Gel offers a nice product for a post-play routine. This pharmacologist-formulated gel is designed to provide instant soothing and cooling relief, helping your tush feel refreshed. It is a hydrogel, similar to what is used in vascular surgery which has been proven to aid in healing and recovery time. If you care enough to moisturize your face after shaving, you should also moisturize your butt after analing.

Believe it or not, there is such a thing as too much lube. If it travels too far into the sigmoid colon, it can stimulate the large intestine, potentially leading to an unexpected and messy situation.

CHAPTER 15

THE MEDICAL SIDE OF PROSTATE PLAY

Overview

- Prostate stimulation supports overall health by supporting prostate function and testosterone levels.
- Prioritize safety by using good hygiene practices, avoiding drugs, and watching for signs of pain or injury.
- Seeking professional guidance can help navigate challenges.
- Don't become an ass junkie and OD on your own dopamine supply.

They say self-care is important—well, this kind of care is next level. Think of prostate stimulation as a biological hack. It can help with several issues, including erectile dysfunction, urinary tract inflammation, and prostate health. It can also combat bladder and fecal incontinence from loss of muscle tone in the pelvic floor.

Your vagus nerve begins in the brain, extends down to the

intestines, and connects with the anus along its path. When you stimulate your ass, you actually activate this nerve, which can help lower your heart rate and blood pressure. Many medical journals have published articles that advocate for prostate massage as a treatment for chronic prostatitis (inflammation of the prostate gland), infertility, benign prostate hypertrophy (BPH), and other sexual problems. Improving prostate health involves actively reducing congested, inflamed, and toxic fluids—a crucial factor in preventing cancer. Prostate stimulation plays a significant role in enhancing overall health and well-being.

> An untreated enlarged prostate can lead to issues like incontinence, and blood in your urine. This is caused by inflammation from straining to pee. See a doctor if you are experiencing any of these symptoms.

Moreover, prostate play eliminates adhesions, and it actively stimulates blood flow, thereby improving circulation. As a result, the prostate receives a greater supply of blood, oxygen, vital nutrients, and white blood cells, thus equipping it to effectively combat infections.

Think of your prostate as a relay system. For instance, a healthy prostate sends signaling messages to the pituitary gland. This complex gland below the brain then sends messages to other glands, such as the adrenal, testicles, thyroid, etc. This helps generate sexual energy, stamina, and even mental clarity. A healthy prostate also helps the testicles manufacture testosterone and sperm. Leaving your prostate without stimulation can cause infection, inflammation, and prostate congestion that can block passages, and cause prostatic fluids to collect. If prostatic fluids are not released, your body becomes an easy target for many microbes, viruses, and yeasts that can harm you. These collected toxic fluids enlarge the prostate. When the prostate is filled with congested fluids, the pituitary gland gets the wrong message and is told to prevent the reproductive process. This results in lower sperm counts, less testosterone, low libido, etc. And it causes you to become weaker, age faster, and gain weight. Start thinking about your prostate as a fountain of youth.

A healthy prostate fosters high levels of testosterone, leading to heightened sexual desire, improved erections, and increased energy. To experience powerful orgasms, the prostate requires unobstructed passages, clear prostatic fluid, and strong muscular contractions.

Regular therapeutic prostate stimulation offers additional benefits by reducing the size of an enlarged prostate, and relieving pressure on the urethra. This restoration of proper bladder function and urine flow rate control is very important. In some traditional Japanese families, wives often engage in prostate massage to promote the health of their husbands, contributing to the lower rates of prostate cancer observed among Asian men when compared to their American counterparts.

Despite doing everything in your power to be healthy, sometimes the prostate will not be receptive to anal play. This can cause frustration for some when trying to attain anal bliss. Psychological trauma (PTSD), drug use, anxiety, ADHD, hormone therapy, autism, depression, schizophrenia, and other factors (e.g., hypertonic pelvic floor condition, TURP surgery to remove parts of the prostate gland through the penis, etc.)

also contribute heavily to the inability to achieve prostate orgasms. The mental health factor is real. Some might also struggle with dysfunction that comes with selective serotonin reuptake inhibitors (SSRIs). This may greatly limit your ability to have a prostate orgasm. Seeking counseling from a doctor can help you better understand the limitations and challenges here.

Safety

Be vigilant for any signs of pain or blood during your prostate play sessions. Each time you insert anything inside you, micro-fissures can occur. These small tears may not initially bleed or cause discomfort, but they can accumulate over time. If you feel pain and spot redness, it's a clear indication that you've either stretched too far or haven't used enough lubrication. Remember the Golden Rule? **Stop when you feel pain!**

An anal fissure is a rectal tear that, although not severe, can take several months to heal. See a doctor, rest, and eat a high-fiber diet to aid in the healing process. If you notice bright red blood without any pain, it's likely a hemorrhoid. This is a common occurrence in individuals who receive anal penetration or strain excessively during bowel movements, such as those with constipation. Hemorrhoids can persist for a prolonged period and may rebleed. But they can also resolve on their own with the use of over-the-counter creams over an extended period. And by staying hydrated!

Engaging in anal play is generally considered safe, as long as the toys used are not abrasive or capable of causing cuts. Additionally, it's important to ensure that the toys are of appropriate size, firmness (not too hard of an object that it tears your skin when you are working it in and out), and length to avoid any potential issues.

To follow are some of the **Basic Safety Rules**:

- Do not mix or use drugs, especially if you have medical prescriptions. Poppers and erection pills are deadly. Again, **never mix them!** CBD and legal weed can be helpful in the right amount. But use caution if you have any medical conditions. Consult a doctor!
- Be hydrated and only play when you are in full health. "Listen" to your body at all times; and stop immediately when you are in any pain.
- Only use toys that have a base at the end. No one wants to visit the emergency room and explain to the doctor that your ass "accidentally fell on a cucumber!"
- Use lots of lube before inserting anything, choose small toys and go shallow at first.
- Play only with clean toys. Neglecting their maintenance can lead to the spread of infections. Before and after each use, it's essential to clean every toy with warm water and soap. For a thorough deep cleaning, don't hesitate to toss them in the dishwasher (no heat) and let it do its work.
- Since the rectum is cellularly engineered to absorb water and anything else it meets, be careful what you put inside you. Like your liver, the rectum will absorb harmful things to filter out toxins. This includes toxic lube and toys. Anything you use for anal play should be composed of ingredients that are safe to consume. That is why many people prefer FDA approved lubes (e.g., "fertility-safe" or "sperm-safe").

Always remember to practice safe sex-toy hygiene!

While prostate massage is beneficial for most, it does come with some risks for certain individuals. These include exacerbating prostatitis, spreading infection leading to sepsis or blood poisoning, triggering cellulitis, causing rectal bleeding, and aggravating hemorrhoids. Furthermore, after drainage, prostate play can result in an amplified burning sensation. **It is important that you consult with your doctor beforehand to discuss the potential risks vs. benefits**.

The anal mucosa, as well as the anus itself, is highly sensitive. While the anus is designed to stretch, it is susceptible to tearing if you are not careful. Reckless anal stimulation can tear your ass and give rise to serious complications that may leave you vulnerable to infections.

Lastly, dopamine is the reward neurotransmitter released when we have an orgasm or are becoming sexually aroused. Too much masturbation (such as ballooning and edging) and anal play leads to way too much dopamine in the brain over time. **Prostrain in moderation**. Otherwise, the brain starts to down-regulate your dopamine system, and this is not good! It causes your body to cease responding to dopamine. Long-term effects can lead to issues like depression, fatigue, cognitive health issues, lack of motivation, and issues with libido and sexual health. Anal orgasms are addictive, so watch for any of these aforementioned signs and discontinue if you see a negative pattern occurring. Please get outside and live a healthy life. Be social, read, exercise and do not spend most of the hours of your week playing with yourself. Life is too beautiful and short to be wasted!

CHAPTER 16

MORE ON PROSTATE HEALTH . . .

Overview

- Prostate exams and a healthy lifestyle support long-term wellness.
- Boost sexual vitality and pleasure with supplements.
- More analogies proving your ass is basically a high-performance vehicle.

Think of your prostate like the oil filter in a car. It might be small and out of sight, but when it's working properly, everything runs smoothly. Ignore it for too long, though, and you could face some serious breakdowns. The stats don't lie: 1 in 8 men will be diagnosed with prostate cancer in their lifetime, and it's the second leading cause of cancer deaths in men. Yet, when detected early, the survival rate is over 99%. That's right—99%! So, why wouldn't you want to have the doctor pop the hood and make sure everything is in top shape?

Let's face it—talking about prostate exams might not be the most exciting topic in this book, but it's essential maintenance.

Skipping out on screenings doesn't make you brave; it just makes you reckless. Men over 50, or even earlier if you have a family history, should be having this conversation with their doctors. PSA tests and screenings are quick, effective, and can literally save your life. It's like having a dashboard warning light—don't wait until smoke is pouring out of the engine to figure out something's wrong.

On top of that, maintaining a healthy lifestyle plays a big role in prostate health. Studies show that regular exercise and a balanced diet rich in fruits, vegetables, and healthy fats can lower your risk. You don't have to become a kale-chomping yoga master (unless you want to), but small changes like cutting back on meat and processed foods, or getting in a brisk walk daily, can make a big difference.

For me, this isn't just about stats or science—it's personal. I get checked regularly because I want to be there for my family when I am older. I don't want to leave my loved ones grieving over something that could have been caught early and treated. I don't want to follow in my dad's footsteps and ignore it. Prostate cancer is beatable when detected in time. So, book that appointment, have the conversation, and take control of your health.

You're not just doing it for yourself—you're doing it for the people who care about you. And it's also a great opportunity to bring up some of the topics from this book and seek your doctor's guidance during your appointment. Why not kill two birds with one dildo and make the most of your visit?

> Get a colonoscopy if you are 45 or older. It's the second-leading cause of cancer deaths in the United States.

Priming the Pump with Supplements

When it comes to boosting sperm production, improving sexual vitality, and enhancing libido, supplements can play a powerful role in complementing both prostate play and a healthy lifestyle. Many vitamins and minerals are directly linked to reproductive health and hormonal balance, which are crucial for optimal sperm quality and quantity (i.e., the more sperm in the reserves, the more intense your prostate orgasms will feel).

Supplements like zinc, selenium, and folic acid have been shown to improve sperm quality as well. Zinc is helpful because it supports testosterone production, a hormone critical for both sperm development and sexual drive. Many herbal supplements also work to improve energy levels and blood circulation, which can directly enhance sexual performance and satisfaction. These natural options provide a holistic approach to enhancing your pleasure.

However, supplements work best when combined with a balanced diet, regular exercise, and stress management. Staying hydrated, maintaining a healthy weight, and limiting exposure to environmental toxins can amplify the benefits of these nutrients, leading to more significant improvements in your overall sexual health.

Always consult a doctor before starting any supplements. Your doctor will be able to ensure they do not interfere with other medications you are taking, and that they do not affect your current health conditions. Here is a list of what I take to "prime the pump" the morning or day before a session:

- **Yohimbine:** Derived from the bark of the Yohimbe tree, this compound is known to improve blood flow and support erectile function by enhancing nitric oxide levels in the body.
- **Saw Palmetto and Pygeum Complex:** A blend of herbal extracts that promote prostate health, reduce inflammation, and support healthy testosterone levels, contributing to better sexual and reproductive function.
- **Maca Extract:** A Peruvian root traditionally used to enhance libido, stamina, and overall energy, while also supporting hormonal balance and sperm quality.
- **L-Tyrosine:** An amino acid that helps produce dopamine and norepinephrine, supporting mood, stress reduction, and sexual desire.
- **L-Arginine and L-Citrulline Complex:** A combination of amino acids that boost nitric oxide production, improving blood circulation and erectile function.
- **Lecithin:** A phospholipid that supports sperm volume and quality, as well as overall cell membrane health.
- **B12 with Folic Acid (Dropper Liquid):** Essential B vitamins that improve red blood cell production, energy metabolism, and sperm DNA integrity, playing a critical role in reproductive health.
- **Muira Puama:** Known as "potency wood", this Amazonian herb enhances sexual desire and helps combat fatigue, promoting overall vitality.
- **Ginseng:** A traditional herbal adaptogen that improves energy, circulation, and stamina, while boosting libido and erectile performance.
- **Tribulus Terrestris Extract:** A natural testosterone

booster that supports sexual function, libido, and fertility of sperm.

- **Ashwagandha:** Reduces stress and anxiety, supports testosterone levels, and enhances overall vitality.
- **Niacin (Vitamin B3):** Promotes better blood flow, reducing vascular issues and enhancing erectile function, while also supporting energy metabolism for overall vitality.

This is a big list, and you do not need to buy or take every single one! Try one at time and see which ones work best for you. More importantly, talk with your doctor to make sure it does not interfere with other medications or health conditions.

This book is shared in honor of the Prostate Cancer Foundation, an organization with an outstanding Charity Navigator rating that advances awareness and research. This cause is deeply personal to me—my father battled prostate cancer before his passing. It's a fight I'm committed to acknowledging. If you take away one thing from this book, let it be the importance of getting screened regularly for prostate cancer. It's one of the most common cancers affecting men, but early detection can make all the difference.

CHAPTER 17

TROUBLESHOOTING

Overview

- Trouble reaching a prostate orgasm could be lack of body awareness, technique issues, or nerve sensitivity.
- Stress, health, and lifestyle factors play a big role—fix these, and progress comes easier.
- Damn, I'm starting to sound like your dad now!

Difficulty in reaching a prostate orgasm can happen due to various reasons. The most common are unfamiliarity with one's own body and lack of knowledge about the prostate's location and sensitivity. This keeps many prostrainers from successfully stimulating the prostate. Inadequate or improper techniques, such as applying too much or too little pressure, or using uncomfortable positions, will also get in the way of progress. Understanding one's body, exploring different techniques patiently, and prioritizing relaxation and comfort are crucial steps toward overcoming these obstacles. If you feel you've tried everything and found nothing that works, take inventory of your situation.

Here are some points I've covered earlier that might be causing blockages:

- The pudendal and perineal nerves extend just outside the scrotum, running from the penile head to the inguinal canal. These nerves form a bundled string between the testicles and legs. The pudendal serves as the primary nerve of the perineum, transmitting sensation from the external genitalia of both sexes, and the skin around the anus and perineum. This is the sweet spot! Additionally, it supplies motor function to various pelvic muscles, including the biological male or female external urethral sphincter and the external anal sphincter. Temporary blockages, as part of a surgery (anesthetic procedure), can also limit the ability to reach anal orgasms.
- Your gut makes most of the body's serotonin, a chemical that affects your mood. The tiny organisms in your gut (called the gut biome) play a role in your overall health and might even block pleasure during prostate play if they're out of balance. This can lead to heightened inflammation and hormonal imbalances, ultimately impairing sexual function.
- Starting with excessive stress can hinder progress in prostate play. Mastery of breathing, relaxation, and mental clarity is crucial. The parasympathetic nervous system (PNS), activated during rest, contrasts the sympathetic nervous system's (SNS) "fight or flight" response. A healthy mind efficiently produces more dopamine and oxytocin, supplementing arousal and interest in sexual activity. If you are facing significant life challenges, achieving prostate orgasms can be challenging. Seeking therapy before resuming practice when ready is advisable.

- Lack of routine or structure, insufficient practice, and understanding that the mind is a powerful sex organ are key aspects. The brain generates pleasure in conjunction with pelvic contractions. Regular practice can lead to experiencing pleasure and orgasms without physical stimulation.
- An untreated enlarged prostate can lead to various health issues. Regular doctor checkups for pain, and understanding the prostate's role as a signaling hub, are essential. A healthy prostate aids in generating sexual energy, stamina, mental clarity, and heightened libido. To experience powerful orgasms, the prostate requires unobstructed passages, clear prostatic fluid, and strong muscular contractions.
- Factors like psychological trauma (PTSD), drug use, anxiety, ADHD, autism, depression, schizophrenia, hypertonic pelvic floor conditions, and effects from selective serotonin reuptake inhibitors (SSRIs) can heavily impact the ability to achieve prostate orgasms.
- Get tested for sexually transmitted infections (STIs). There's no direct, well-established evidence that STIs specifically affect prostate orgasms, but they can influence prostate health and sexual function more broadly. This might indirectly impact the experience specifically affect prostate orgasms. For example, bacterial STIs can spread to the prostate, causing acute or chronic prostatitis. Symptoms like pain, swelling, or irritation could make prostate stimulation uncomfortable or less enjoyable, potentially diminishing the intensity of a prostate orgasm. Non-bacterial STIs, like herpes or HPV, don't directly target the prostate

but could affect overall pelvic health or sexual comfort, indirectly influencing the experience.

- Previous surgeries, particularly those involving the spine or areas near the reproductive and urogenital systems, can impact sensitivity and nerve
- Excessive play can lead to desensitization and damage to the rectum; also consider that hemorrhoids will cause discomfort and make it difficult to feel pleasure.
- Unhealthy weight gain can pose additional challenges. Strengthening core muscles and maintaining a healthy lifestyle can aid in proficiency with anal orgasms.

Talk with your doctor or therapist if any of these concerns might be an issue for you. And return to your journey once (and if) you overcome these challenges.

Here's a handy checklist that captures most everything we'll cover in the book. Bring it along to your next doctor's visit and feel free to discuss anything on the list that's on your mind. Your doctor is likely much more approachable than you might expect! Don't worry about being judged — there's no need to hold back.

Doctor Checklist

☐ Safely stretching and stimulating the prostate?
☐ Numbing cream for first time?
☐ SSRIs and prostate play.
☐ Anal fissure or rectal tears.
☐ Discuss any blood in stool or urine, straining to pee, hemorrhoids or any other current health issues.
☐ CBD/THC, drug interactions and medical conditions.

☐ Prostate cancer & colonoscopy screenings?

☐ Supplements and health conditions?

☐ E-stim, penis pumps, percussion guns, sex machines?

☐ Stress, health, and lifestyle factors?

☐ PTSD, STIs, previous surgeries, mental health, etc.

CHAPTER 18

BALLOONING AND EDGING TECHNIQUES

Overview

- Edging and ballooning can intensify anal orgasms, unlocking deeper sensations.
- These techniques help build arousal and prolong pleasure for stronger releases.
- Innovative ways to achieve the finest case of blue balls.

Edging creates intense arousal. It involves stimulating your penis until the "edge of cumming", then holding yourself back from ejaculating. Ballooning is similar; however, it requires more self-discipline and is an advanced method of edging. In short, ballooning discourages the stimulation of the sensitive parts of the penis (frenulum and head).

Both are like standing at the crest of a roller coaster, teetering just before the drop. You feel the rush building, the anticipation rising, and every second you hold off makes the eventual plunge even more exhilarating. It's all about savoring the suspense and amplifying the thrill before letting yourself freefall into pure bliss.

Remember: If you edge (or balloon) and want intense anal orgasms, then do not ejaculate! With practice, you can build up a rhythm and have an almost endless string of anal orgasms, once you learn your preferred technique and style.

Ballooning

Think of it as a great exercise in self-control. Ballooning requires you to become sexually aroused and erect to an extreme without overstimulating your nervous system. This helps to stop the flood of noradrenaline, adrenaline, and cortisone. You massage only the nerves on the "belly side" of the penis (underneath side), focusing on the sensation of your orgasmic energy. The focus here should be breathing into the diaphragm and anus area (anal "breathing") when doing this. Sessions usually last between 30-60 minutes. How do you do this? Good question.

1. Ballooning should be done lying down.
2. Relax all your muscles so that the only thing moving is your hand rubbing the underneath of your cock, scrotum, and perineum.
3. Give attention to each area of these genital areas. The base and shaft, the scrotum and the pubis area of the groin, should all be vigorously worked with hands and fingers.
4. It is highly recommended that you perform reverse kegels at the same time. Take a deep breath from your diaphragm, hold your reverse kegels for at least 5 seconds to allow your pelvic floor muscles to build

arousal. Then release your breath deeply and begin another reverse kegel.

5. Find a rhythm to your breath to follow the rhythm of your kegels. Remember, only stroke your lower shaft (above your testes) and the perineum. Rub that perineum upwards like you are doing a come hither with three fingers (imagine it is a pussy and you are rubbing it upwards). Do not touch your penis head, as tempting as it will be.

6. Continue short reverse kegels while rubbing yourself. You should get harder and more aroused.

7. **Pay attention to the levels of arousal as you build close to orgasm.** Try to imagine each one and the feelings you experience during each level.

8. When you feel like you are about to orgasm, slow down and do more short reverse kegels to let your body cool down.

9. Restart the process when you feel like you are no longer near a level 9.5 arousal level. Repeat for around 30-60 minutes and try to get to 3-5 near-orgasms in a session.

10. Also, when you feel like you are about to reach Level 9.5-9.9, now squeeze the tip of the penis very hard with your fingers (almost painfully) and do a strong reverse kegel to stop the orgasm. This will better help you from going over the edge.

11. After you get better at this, do ballooning with frenulum play; aka, just rubbing the penis head glands. See how far you can go without cumming.

12. Repeat 3 to 5 times a week.

Once you learn to control the ejaculation, the spongy tissues of the organ become more flexible and conditioned. This helps with building blood circulation and muscle control. The technique will grow your penis to maximum length/girth and even gives you stronger erections. Ballooning can be a highly rewarding technique, especially while doing your kegel routines. But it takes time to master.

Edging

Edging is much different than ballooning. You use your standard masturbation techniques (direct gland stroking stimulation), get to a Level 9 arousal level, then stop. You stay between a Level 5 arousal, then go back to Level 9, over and over for an hour or more.

There are many ways you can practice edging orgasm control techniques. Figure out what works best for you by experimenting with different ones.

Edging and ballooning can be a highly useful exploration, bringing your awareness to your arousal, and experimenting with what it feels like to ride that edge of climax. For both of these techniques, you can use hands or toys to explore. **The key is to go slowly and deliberately, paying attention to your body's arousal signals and levels.** Mindfully notice each one, and the feelings and emotions you experience during each level.

Never let your orgasm take over! When you get to that Level 9 arousal, squeeze the head of your penis so no semen escapes. Stop and hold the squeeze for at least 30 seconds or until the pulsing and throbbing stops. Afterward, breathe deeply and run your hands over your nipples and other parts of your body. Let your body enjoy this incredible heightened arousal.

Think about what brought you close to orgasm, and take mental notes on how your body feels. This will help when you move to anal orgasm play afterward. Doing either ballooning or edging before anal play will drive your arousal to new levels, and help you achieve intense anal orgasms. Incorporating kegel exercises at the peak of your arousal can unlock entirely new dimensions of sensation and discovery.

> **Pro Tip**: Set up your anal play routine before edging/ballooning. Do everything you need to do (douching, emptying your bladder, etc.) so you can transition quickly to anal play after a good edging/ballooning session. This helps you get closer to reaching anal orgasms, Super-Os, etc. Also, practice edging using a toy (sex machine preferably). When you get to an arousal level of 9-9.5, stop edging and use your anal play skills to send you over the edge hands-free.

Repeat as often as you like. Here is where you'll plunge deep into the art of bridging the gap between the two types of orgasms and mastering the techniques for achieving a hands-free orgasm.

CHAPTER 19

THE BEST POSITIONS FOR PROSTATE ORGASMS

Overview

- Discover the best positions to maximize prostate stimulation and pleasure.
- Learn how angles, pillows, and body alignment enhance sensation.
- The perfect angle is like tuning a radio—move around until you hit the right frequency.

Good penetration can provide multi-sensory arousal to all the erogenous zones of your body. This is another piece of the puzzle you will need to figure out during prostate play.

Arching the back while trying to clench during kegels makes it somewhat easier to isolate the right muscles and not activate the sphincter. Everyone is different. Explore and find what works best for your body type. I recommend using pillows for different angles and getting creative as possible. Watching videos of others having hands-free orgasms is a good way to learn new positions as well. **Reddit** and **RedGifs** have a decent collection throughout the subreddits (e.g., **reddit.com/r/CumFromAnal** or **redgifs.com/gifs/hands-free**). But there are plenty of free "tube" sites if you do a search with terms such as: hands-free orgasm, prostate orgasms, or sissygasm.

Also check out **Xvideos, PornHub,** and any other popular, adult-streaming site.

For many prostrainers, missionary, lying on the side, and doggy style are the standard for prostate play. I recommend, however, that you explore the following yoga poses after you get more comfortable with your practice. Do not enter any position if you feel pain or are using your muscles uncomfortably to maintain a pose. Your poses should be relaxing and calm. **Speak to a medical professional about which of the following poses might exacerbate existing back, hip, or other musculoskeletal issues.** And be sure to use pillows and cushions for support, so you are not exerting your muscles.

Bridge Pose

- Lie on your back.
- Bend both knees and position your feet hip-width apart with knees in line with ankles. Feet are on the floor.
- Put your arms flat on the floor with palms against the ground and spread your fingers.
- Lift your pelvic region off the ground (use a pillow or yoga block to support your spine), allowing your torso to follow; but keep your shoulders and head on the floor.

Happy Baby

- Lie on your back.
- With an exhale, bend knees up toward your stomach.
- Inhale and reach up to grab the outside of your feet, then widen your knees. You can also use a belt or towel looped over your foot to make it easier. Or, if you have a sex swing (or yoga swing) ceiling mount, use it to offset gravity, utilizing the straps to keep your feet in the air.
- Flex your feet, pushing heels upward as you pull down with your hands to stretch.

Child's Pose

- Start by kneeling on the floor. With your big toes touching, widen your knees until they're around hip-width apart.
- Exhale and lean forward. Place your hands in front of you and stretch out, allowing your upper body to relax between your legs. Try to touch your forehead to the mat, but you can also rest your head on a block or pillow.
- Relax in this position and melt away.

Boat Pose

- Sit on the floor with knees bent.
- Clasp knees with hands and lean back onto the floor.
- Squeeze the muscles of your hips and abdomen while keeping your chest high and your body still.
- As you hold this position, inhale to stretch your spine, and exhale to tighten your core.

Fetal Pose

- Lie on your back.
- Turn to one side. Extend the bottom arm and bend the knees. Rest your head on your arm with legs bent.
- Keep your eyes closed.
- Try this pose and add some movement as if you are climbing a rope or pole. This can elevate arousal.

Standing Position

- Stand up straight and spread your legs. Put the toy or machine underneath.
- Bend knees a little to find your comfort zone. Your knees will project a little out over your feet, and your trunk can lean slightly forward over thighs. Play and find the best center of gravity for you.
- It is best if you can grab onto something like a bar or rope. If you have a yoga swing ceiling mount, use it to offset gravity.

Garland or Squat Pose

- Squat down. Keep heels on the floor if you can, otherwise, support them on a folded mat.
- Separate thighs slightly wider than your torso.
- Press hands or elbows on knees. This will help lengthen your front torso. Like standing position, this pose tends to hit the prostate perfectly.

Whatever position you choose, practice crossing your legs

and spreading them wider, lifting them, etc. Sometimes making these adjustments activates the prostate in ways that you never would have imagined.

In addition to investing in a yoga swing ceiling mount or a sex swing, I highly recommend adding a wedge pillow to your collection—it's a game-changer. Some wedge pillows even come with printed sex position cards to spark inspiration and creativity.

Also, try a suction-cup dildo in the shower. Attach it to a wall and go at it. A very relaxing and enjoyable experience with the hot water running. **Try to aim for an angle that points toward your stomach.** This typically feels best, and it makes sense anatomically when placing pressure on your prostate.

The positions below illustrate a few varieties that you can experiment with. Some are similar to the yoga positions previously mentioned. Play around with all of them to find the right angle for you. Use pillows or furniture to get the best angle. Practice makes perfect!

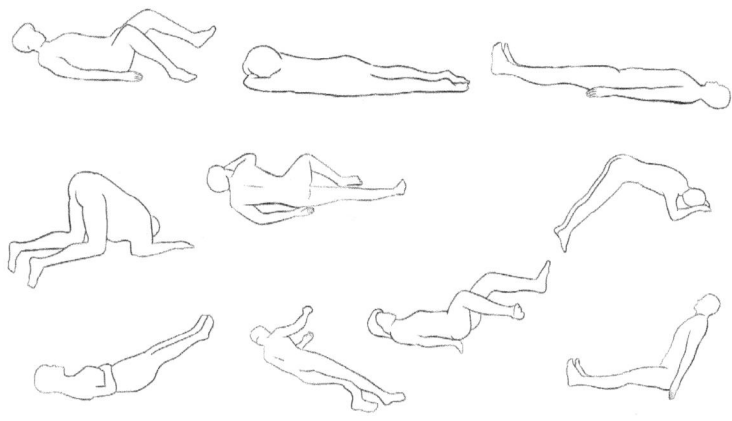

Find the best position that matches your ability and comfort. Modify as needed. Find a partner to help if possible.

Honorable mention: Try the pile driver position. Lie on your back, take a bunch of pillows or a wedge pillow so your butt is lifted as high as possible. You can also use a yoga sling or sex swing that lets your legs rise high, so the sex machine can drill that prostate. Legs can be moved between 45 and 90 degrees. Once you find that sweet spot, there's no going back. Lying on your back with your feet up the wall, you move between quick thrusts and longer strokes until you reach the point where it feels like you have to pee. As you relax, you keep applying pressure with the tip of your toy against the prostate until fluids shoot out. You also discover the art of timing and positions—when to clench differently, when to adjust for the right angle, when to allow the pressure to build, and when to simply relax and let the orgasms flow.

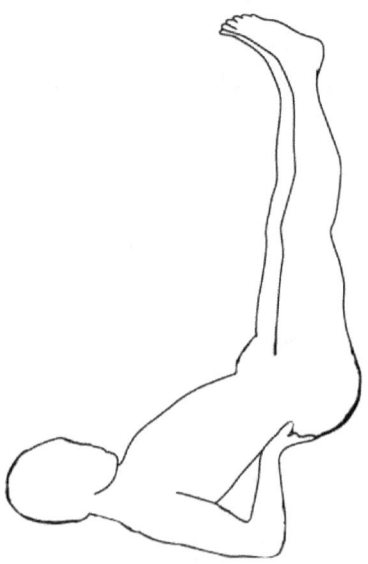

CHAPTER 20

CHEMICAL ENHANCEMENTS

Overview

- Drugs can disrupt natural pleasure responses, impair judgment, and pose serious health risks.
- Apologies for the buzzkill—I'm your high school guidance counselor now.

Drugs affect prostate play in many ways. They can increase or decrease libido and sexual response, making sexual pleasure more or less intense. Often, the effects of drugs are unpredictable. A drug that has a positive effect one day, could easily produce a negative effect the next time. Never combine prescription and recreational drugs; this can have serious consequences.

BE AWARE: Know your state drug laws and consult a doctor before you even consider these options. There are many areas of caution, ranging from dosage to setting, current health complications, etc. A person should be in a positive headspace, and a safe environment, before using anything that will disrupt your natural mood.

Weed and CBD: CBD helps reduce anxiety, increase lubrication, and relax muscles. It is often used for anal play. Both weed (THC) and CBD can help get you in the right mood. CBD increases blood flow to tissues in reproductive organs and sexual tissue. Studies have shown cannabis may be helpful for people with a low sex drive.

Fortunately, mild use of CBD or THC has no serious known side effects and is unlikely to be fatal when used correctly. Nevertheless, discuss with a healthcare professional before using any form of cannabis. If you choose to use THC, start with a small dosage. Many prostate enthusiasts report that strains high in terpene linalool enhance prostate play due to its calming effect. Weed and CBD can also have a laxative effect prior to anal play. This will make it more likely that you might have fecal secretions during your sessions when you use these products. Make sure to avoid eating a big meal within a few hours of when you plan to play; and flush (enema, douches, etc.) out everything thoroughly prior to using weed and CBD.

Different strains of cannabis produce different results. Indica strains give you a body high and make everything in your body very sensitive. Sativa strains also produce very euphoric results, making your orgasms feel warm, tingly, with feelings of happiness and joy. Some anal enthusiasts will combine both strains for longer, more intense sessions. **Always use caution if you decide to experiment with these drugs**.

! WARNING: I PERSONALLY DO NOT USE
OR RECOMMEND ANY OF THE FOLLOWING
DRUGS. I AM LISTING THEM TO GIVE YOU
A HEADS-UP ON THE POSSIBLE ADVERSE
SIDE EFFECTS. I STRONGLY SUGGEST YOU
CONSULT WITH, AND GET AN OKAY FROM,
YOUR PHYSICIAN BEFORE EXPERIMENTING
WITH ANY OF THEM!

Erectile dysfunction (ED) Drugs: Prescribed ED medications (known as phosphodiesterase type 5 PDE5 inhibitors) work by relaxing the smooth muscle in the blood vessels inside your penis. While most are generally safe and effective, they can have side effects, such as headaches, nasal congestion, and visual disturbances. In some rare cases, they can cause severe side effects, like hearing or vision loss, priapism (a prolonged and painful erection), and other strong allergic reactions. Never mix these with poppers—the result can be fatal!

Poppers: Often marketed as "VCR head cleaner", this chemical liquid makes penetration feel like an orgasm. It's a vasodilator that opens up your blood vessels; and causes a dip in blood pressure, followed by warm, fuzzy feelings. Your heart rate spikes to maintain normal blood pressure, and you rush off into space for a few minutes.

Poppers enhance play sessions by enhancing your tactical senses. They also cause you to simultaneously relax and put you into a dirty slut mode. Poppers may help with relaxing the sphincter, but don't experiment with them when you are stretching; otherwise, you might hurt/tear yourself.

Study the types available and choose the brand carefully. Stay away from Isopropyl Nitrite, as it can damage your vision. The better ones are Isoamyl Nitrite, Isobutyl Nitrite, and n-butyl Nitrite. But all poppers can cause serious side effects, such as low blood oxygen and even death. Poppers quickly wear off, and you return to the level you were at before you inhaled, sometimes feeling a loss of arousal, headache, etc. I repeat: **Never mix poppers with ED drugs—or the results can be fatal!** Also, do not combine poppers with any medicine or vitamins that reduce blood pressure. Never allow poppers to come in contact with the mouth, eyes, or mucus membranes. **Again, I highly recommend NOT using poppers.**

Entheogens: Psilocybin/LSD, and/or MDMA can be one of the most intense experiences during penetration. **At the same time, it can be one of the most dangerous chemical enhancements to experiment with during prostate play.** Some have found that LSD with MDMA produce the most orgasmic sessions. Mushrooms are said to be very different and veer you into an unexpected realm.

Overall, these substances have a high probability of leading to intense physical and mystical experiences. Studies have shown they may reduce or eliminate anxiety and distress, while increasing openness, e.g., the capacity for fantasy, appreciation of new feelings/sensations and increased tolerance levels. The downside: Loss of concentration during anal play and the possibility of a "bad trip". As many advise, you should be in a positive headspace and a safe environment before using psychedelics.

And I repeat: I highly recommend NOT using these drugs.

CHAPTER 21

MINDGASM VERSUS A-LESS

Overview

- Compare Mindgasm (mental orgasms) with (anal stimulation-free) techniques.
- Explore how mental focus and physical engagement create different orgasmic experiences.
- Learn A-less techniques to achieve prostate orgasms.
- In a sea of dildos, suffering from the thrust of penetrations and the rattling of vibrations, there is solace for some in the world of A-less or Mindgasm.

This is a short introduction to these practices. An entire book could be written for each one. As you become more proficient in prostate play, I recommended that you explore each of these worlds. Many experienced prostrainers view the use of toys with prostate stimulation as training wheels. Some hold the opinion that you can experience deeper, more meaningful prostate orgasms by using only the power of your mind to control your body, rather than relying on toys to enhance arousal.

I personally believe the answer is in the middle of these two realms. And ultimately, it just depends on your personality, mood for the day, and overall preference.

Mental orgasms are linked to the neuroplexus—a complex network of nerves and vessels within your body. Often called a vagus nerve orgasm, they share similarities with the cervical orgasm. This type of climax involves a profound release of tension deep within the abdomen, creating a sensation that feels like a slow, volcanic eruption in the belly. As it builds and releases, the pleasure radiates outward, engulfing the entire body in waves of euphoria. Some say it feels like taking MDMA or DMT (i.e., synthetic psychedelic drugs that cause feelings of love and oneness)!

You will see the words Mindgasm and A-less pop up in the prostate play community. In short, Mindgasm is a formal program that takes more of a mental approach to pleasure, while teaching various pelvic floor exercise techniques. **A-less focuses on engaging the body through physical techniques such as controlled pelvic floor muscle contractions** (like kegels) and mindful breathing exercises. The primary difference between the two lies in their focus. A-less is rooted in physical stimulation and control, requiring a strong awareness of, and connection to, the pelvic floor muscles to achieve prostate pleasure. In contrast, **Mindgasm centers on mental techniques, relying on the brain's ability to generate sensations through visualization and focus.** Both methods are complementary and offer unique pathways to pleasure—one through mastering the body—and the other through harnessing the mind. Together, they provide a holistic approach to exploring new dimensions of sexual fulfillment.

A-less and Mindgasm are like two paths up the same mountain, each offering a unique journey to the summit of pleasure.

A-less is the rugged, hands-on climb. You're engaging your body, feeling the terrain underfoot, and using physical strength and technique to ascend. It's about mastering the tools you already have—your pelvic floor muscles, breathing, and body awareness—to navigate the journey. Each step builds a direct, visceral connection with the experience, making the climb itself as rewarding as reaching the peak. You are alone the whole time and there is no designated path up.

Mindgasm, on the other hand, is the scenic gondola ride. Instead of relying on physical effort, you're letting your mind guide you effortlessly through the heights of pleasure. Visualization, focus, and mental energy create the experience, allowing you to savor the view from a more abstract and meditative perspective. It's about trusting the power of your imagination and neural pathways to take you where you want to go. Your guide is always there giving you a tour.

Both paths lead to the same destination, but the choice is yours: Do you want to immerse yourself in the physical journey? Or let your mind take the reins? Either way, the summit promises a breathtaking experience.

Mindgasm Explained

In the beginning, this program uses specific kegel exercises to strengthen the pelvic floor muscles, while incorporating musical cues and guided voice narration. It is a structured curriculum containing lessons that provide you with a helpful road map to increase involuntary contractions and learn to achieve the different types of anal orgasms. Mindgasm also takes a more mental approach to pleasure. This technique uses visualization, relaxation, and mental focus to create orgasmic sensations, sometimes without any physical stimulation at all. By leveraging the brain's ability to mimic physical sensations, Mindgasm taps into neural pathways associated with arousal and pleasure. It combines mindfulness, breathwork, and guided imagery to activate the body's pleasure centers, often resulting in what's described as "full-body orgasms."

Ultimately as you progress, the experience is less about engaging the prostate or pelvic floor directly, and more about using the power of the mind to evoke intense sensations. It is a fun, regimented journey that integrates everything you need to leverage the connection between the brain and the body. This program prepares you to experience "energetic orgasms" and discover how to build "waves of pleasure" that flow and radiate throughout your entire body.

Of course, this experience varies for everyone, and some parts of Mindgasm may not be right for you. Either way, I recommended that you do a 30-day trial. This way, you will learn what to incorporate into your routines, and what to discard. For me, it provided a consistent way to get over the learning hump and have regular hands-free wet and Super-O orgasms.

Mindgasm is a well-designed system. As you modify and combine what you learn, you might even find some parts of it are in contradiction to what feels good. Therefore, be flexible and adaptive with it to get the most gains. If you go the full length of their training series—which I highly recommend— you will eventually be able to do many of the activities with only your mind. Check out **mindgasm.net** for more details.

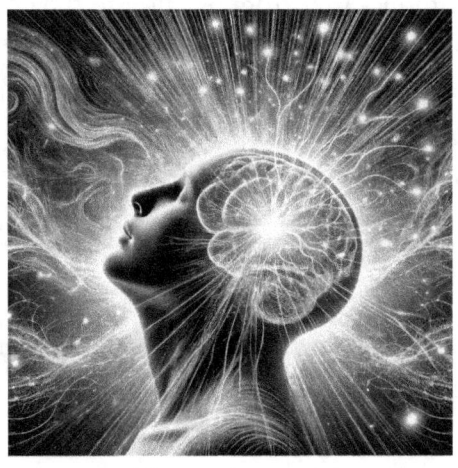

A-Less Explained

A-less (aka "Anerosless", "A-less", "Toy-less", etc.) is where you have any type of prostate orgasm(s) without an Aneros . . . or another instrument inserted inside your ass.

A-less is the graduate school of anal orgasms. A-less focuses on using techniques like intentional muscle contractions, controlled breathing, and mental focus to stimulate the prostate and build arousal. This practice requires patience and practice, as it involves tuning into subtle sensations and learning to control the pelvic floor muscles. Many who explore A-less describe it as a deeply connected and intimate experience, offering a unique way to enhance pleasure while developing greater awareness of the body's capabilities.

A-less techniques vary from one user to the next; and many are homegrown, do-it-yourself methods that stimulate prostate pleasure and various orgasm types. There are not many programs within this realm, outside of a few community forums with shared routines and practices. Even on these sites, there are many differences, beliefs, paths, etc. Like a religion, you have your self-glorified prophets and your casual followers.

A-less is the deepest rabbit hole of prostate play that borders on the realm of spiritual singularity—a universal healing energy flowing into the body and soul that results in full body twisting, and multiple orgasms while glowing in radiant energy. Conversely, sometimes mild A-less orgasms involuntarily occur just sitting in your chair at work. With that said, I recommend you start with an open mind and test-drive the many recommended techniques you can find online as you rewire to this mysterious frequency.

Those who practice A-less often describe it as a journey of discovery. The sensations can range from subtle tingles to powerful, wave-like orgasms that radiate throughout the entire body. These orgasms are less about physical release and more about sustained, whole-body pleasure, leaving many feeling both energized and deeply satisfied.

For background, many start off using an Aneros toy *before* they go to A-less. And once they find out that they can have orgasms with the Aneros, they realize they can have these powerful orgasms without it (thus the term "Aneros-less" = A-less).

An A-less session can go on for hours. It's very convenient with no messy lubes. And once you start, it might become your go-to, leaving your dildos and other toys collecting dust.

A-less is typically enhanced with your body awareness, including deep, rhythmic breathing with relaxed, energetic concentration. It is steered less by your kegels, and best with nipple play. Prostrainers typically go to A-less when they move past penetrative states and transcend into a meditative state of anal orgasms. It is the monastery and nirvana of ass play.

You mentally use both the penis and ass, in terms of pleasure, but the mental focus seeks to unite the neuroplexus (a branching network of vessels and nerves) in your body with your sweet spot of pleasure.

In my experience, A-less is more challenging. It focuses on mindful edging meditation with techniques to move energy and pleasure away from the cock and prostate to the rest of the body's sexual channels. The goal is not to have hands-free wet orgasm (HFWO), though some do. It is more about creating a circulation of Super-Os and tantric sexual energy.

> "The best way to enjoy your job is to imagine yourself without one." — Oscar Wilde

For me, A-less begins with slowing down time and tuning into the deep sexual relaxation. I lie on my back, close my eyes and stretch out my legs, slightly bowing my knees with pillows underneath them. I go very slow with a little "mental" nipple play at first and focus on relaxing my nipples and prostate area as much as possible until involuntary contractions form. I do not let my pelvic floor muscles tighten while I am doing this. I focus my attention on all the areas that feel good (anus, perineum, frenulum, scrotum, base of the penis, etc.). I ride out these tingling feelings and let the P-Waves form.

Usually, my body quivers and the feelings keep intensifying. I focus on the center of this pleasure and let it grow. Often, the pleasure radiates out from genital areas into my heart, legs, fingers, and crown of my head. When I'm lucky, I can keep this feedback loop going, while having precum form. This causes pressure on my bladder; but it's not an uncomfortable feeling, more of an orgasmic wave that forms but never really crashes. This goes on and on until I start having shaking Super-Os, and then it just shuts off for me. Sometimes it ends with some personal enlightenment, much like I get from holotropic breathwork.

Check out the Aneros Forum at **community.aneros.com/ forum**. Also browse, Reddit Communities like **r/ProstatePlay** and **r/SexOver30** for discussions on A-less, including advice and success stories.

A-Less Exercises to Experiment With

These suggested techniques might require a few tryouts. Do not get frustrated if you feel nothing at first. Come back again and again. Once you rewire, these will become easier. And as you master your orgasms, you will be able to fully enjoy the A-less experience. To be more effective, do one or all of them daily for two weeks. Best performed with an empty bladder. Do it in a dark room, use an essential oil scent diffuser, listen to meditation sounds, or anything else that can set the mood and quiet your mind. (Optional: Feel free to use an Aneros at first when learning to master these techniques; eventually practicing without it over time.)

These exercises can stimulate your endocrine system, boosting your virility and sensuality, while transforming bottled-up sexual tension into a state of relaxed and focused pleasure. Feel free to modify them to your liking.

Easy Sunrise

This is both the easiest one and very effective, if you can get relaxed and stay focused on your breath. Using a prostate toy with a sound meditation can bring slow, rising orgasms. Find a long theta or yoga nidra mediation on a video streaming site or meditation app, and listen to it while doing the following:

- Find the best position that feels most pleasurable to you. I prefer lying on my back with a pillow under the legs.
- Start diaphragm breathing, taking long inhales and long exhales. Hold for 3 seconds in between each inhale and exhale.
- Keep taking the deepest breaths possible. While inhaling, squeeze your A-Muscle. When you reach the top of your breath, hold for 3 seconds. Then exhale and do a reverse kegel with your A-Muscle on the breath down, holding for 3 seconds after you fully exhale. Do this for 15-30 minutes and you can start to have several types of prostate orgasms. Increase the level of each squeeze every 2-5 minutes to raise the intensity.
- When the orgasms start coming, incorporate the pulses using your P-Muscle and T-Muscle, if you can. Feel free to incorporate the other pelvic floor region exercises from Chapter 6.

Electric Butterfly Waves

- Begin naked on your back (or any other comfortable position).
- Start with a gentle, light reverse kegel anal contraction (push out), just above the level of relaxing your sphincter.
- Focus on your erogenous zones (penis head, inside thighs, stomach, nipples, etc.) with your hands lightly touching these areas. If you wish, use porn to start your arousal process.
- Inhale deeply, expanding into the lower diaphragm (area below the navel), and vibrate the diaphragm as if sobbing, or catching several mini breaths as you exhale.
- Hold your breath for about 15 seconds, while also crunching down on your abdomen and anus. Do not hold your breath too long and pass out.
- Repeat the inhalation breathing technique making sure you keep a reverse kegel and ab squeeze (extend your belly). As you get more comfortable with maintaining this, slowly increase the kegel contraction to a low-moderate level for a few seconds, then return to the level you started with in the beginning. You are creating a wave pattern here. Experiment with different combinations of breathing, gentle anal contractions, and building an orgasmic wave. Repeat as many of these waves as you can.
- Look for pleasurable electric tingles and butterfly sensations in the stomach. Increase the waves of pleasure in the areas that become activated. Find sensations you have felt before in the areas around your genitals,

abdomen, tailbone, etc.
- As the pleasure grows stronger, concentrate on your prostate area. Concentrate on the area where your pleasure feels most intense and originates. You will start to feel P-Waves, and may even experience anal orgasms.

Extended Male Deer (Tantra Qi Gong practice)

Begin naked either in a chair or on your back in bed. Smile and breathe deeply from your diaphragm. Keep your tongue slightly up in your mouth so the tip is touching the roof. There are two phases to this exercise:

- **Focused body massage:** Warm your hands first and cup your right hand around your testicles. If you can reach, use the right-hand thumb and rest it on top of your penis, gently sandwiching your thumb and penis onto your pubic bone so there is medium to firm pressure. You want to lightly push down, adding pressure on your testicles as well. Now, take the rest of your right-hand fingers and add pressure to your perineum like you are pulling it upwards. Now, take your left hand and place the entire palm just below your belly button (3-4 finger widths). Circle the left hand around this area gently rubbing above your penis shaft. Do this about 100 times (or roughly 2 minutes). Then switch hands and create the circles in the reverse order. Your choice of direction for each hand does not matter, just make sure you go both clockwise and counterclockwise for each one. Let the sensations build. You will experience a soothing, warm sensation flowing up and down your spine. Stay erect during this practice. If you lose your erection, stimulate yourself back to hardness, and return to rubbing.

- **Kegel**: Next, intertwine your fingers and place them in your lap. While you breathe deeply in and out, begin a P-Muscle Kegel. Hold as long as possible, at least 1 minute. Keep your ass and stomach muscles relaxed as you do this kegel. Feel the connection of all of your pleasure areas merge as you hold, letting the sexual energy build in one place.

As you master this exercise, modify the massage part by moving your hands up and down across the top half of your body. Begin above your pubic bone and move up toward your belly with each circle. Go higher up your torso, to the sternum, chest, and neck; then slowly go back down again. You are looking to create a circulation of Super-Os and tantric sexual energy that grows stronger and stronger.

Pulse & Ripple

- Begin naked, resting on your back (or any other comfortable position) in bed, and take several deep breaths.
- If you wish, use porn to start your arousal process. Get yourself primed so you enter this practice at an arousal Level of 7 or higher. Edge or balloon beforehand.
- Close your eyes and tune into the sensations in your body for 2 minutes. Keep breathing deeply and calmly from your diaphragm.
- Squeeze your T-Muscle as lightly as possible. Wait for the slight pulsations to build. You can play with your nipples, but do not stimulate your penis anymore! As

the pleasure rises, lightly squeeze your P-Muscle and A-Muscle, so you are now holding all 3 at the same time. You are looking to create a medium sensation of pleasure (Level 5 arousal). Not too strong or too weak. Remember to keep your breathing steady. When you get to this level, immediately go to the next step . . .

- Quickly stop all the squeezing of your muscles and relax your entire body. **This is the most important step in this exercise**. Do not move, just relax! Keep the breath steady, and feel free to continue playing with your nipples; this will bring deeper states of pleasure, and increased blood flow. Concentrate on the tingling ripple and pulsations of electricity between your legs, around your genital areas, across your stomach, chest and beyond. Feel it spread all over your body. After the sensations reach full intensity, let them wash over you, feeling the waves of orgasms ripple across your body until there is no pleasure left to experience. (This step requires you to use your breath to keep things building. The goal is to take yourself from a Level 5 arousal to a Level 9.5 and beyond.)
- Repeat the cycle as much as you'd like, and until you no longer feel heightened arousal.

Up Down

- Begin naked on your back (or any other comfortable position) in bed and breathe deeply.
- If you wish, use porn to start your arousal process. Get yourself primed so you enter this practice at an arousal Level of 7 or higher. Edge or balloon beforehand.

- Close your eyes and tune into the sensations in your body for 2 minutes. Begin breathing deeply and calmly from your diaphragm.
- Imagine a glowing sexual energy forming around your groin and stomach area. Focus on it and imagine it growing, getting stronger.
- Lightly begin a reverse kegel squeezing your A-Muscle (remember, reverse kegels act as if you are trying to squeeze out poop). Hold your kegel as lightly as possible to a low level for at least 10 seconds. Keep breathing deeply and regularly. Do not hold your breath.
- Lightly begin a regular kegel squeezing your A-Muscle (remember, a regular kegel acts as if you are trying to hold in a fart or keeping your toy from coming out of your ass). Hold your kegel as lightly as possible to a low level for at least 10 seconds. Keep breathing deeply and regularly. Do not hold your breath.
- Repeat these for 2-5 minutes. You can raise the level of intensity of each kegel to moderate, or even high if you can handle it.
- Next, you are going to keep doing the same thing, but in shorter intervals, and keeping the intensity of the squeeze at moderate or high. You want to hold the reverse kegel for 3 seconds, and quickly start a regular kegel for 3 seconds, with no resting in between. The goal is to create a wave pattern.
- Light pulsations generally build rapidly, leading to P-Gasms and Super-Os the longer you go. You can play with your nipples, but do **not** stimulate your penis. As the pleasure starts rising, you can incorporate your T-Muscle and P-Muscle to be creative and

build some pulsing. Remember to keep your breathing steady. Adapt it as you see fit, and follow what works for your body.

The A-less possibilities are endless! Explore, create, and experiment with techniques that resonate with your body. **Think of it like having your own rollercoaster park—you're in control of creating the twists, turns, and climbs, building anticipation and savoring every moment before the ultimate release.** The beauty of A-less lies in its deeply personal nature—there's no right or wrong way to approach it. Embrace the adventure, celebrate the discoveries, and let yourself be amazed by the thrilling ride of unlocking your body's full potential for exhilarating pleasure and connection.

CHAPTER 22

ANAL ORGASMS AND SEXUAL INTER-COURSE

Overview

- Explore the connection between anal orgasms, sexual intercourse, and pegging.
- Learn how communication enhances comfort, trust, and pleasure.
- Read real conversations that bring these experiences to life.
- Not propaganda to take a real dick in your butt . . . unless you're already into that.

There are two ways to have anal orgasms during sex: being a bottom (getting pegged or taking cock) or topping (doing the penetration on someone). First, let's start with topping . . .

The next time you have sex and top, revamp your ordinary sex experience by using anal toys. Experiment with a prostate toy or butt plug—vibrating or non-vibrating. Your erection will be super hard, and your orgasm will be more intense, lasting much longer. These toys will exert heightened pressure on your prostate gland, delivering a surge of stimulation. The feelings of anal contractions will be amplified when you ejaculate. And, if you are lucky, you might even experience anal orgasms before your penile orgasm.

Before starting, secure your anal toy to keep it from popping out of your ass. Remember to go slow and focus on incorporating your PAT method kegels at every stage of sex. **Start with foreplay and build up your arousal.** During penetration, the feeling becomes so much more intense and fun. Your partner will feel it as well when you kegel and clench your anal toy. Let the P-Waves keep building and building while you combine slow breathing into your thrusting. If you are an advanced prostrainer, you'll be able to create a cycle of building anal orgasms, and even Super-Os.

> Anal sex is like a comedy show at a BBQ—it's all about timing, delivery, knowing your audience . . . and having lots of wipes on hand!

The key is to practice regularly, relax deeply, and concentrate on the moment (being present and tuning into each other's sexual energy). The sensations will follow as your arousal builds. Syncing up breathing and muscle contractions with your partner will help the experience. Let your fantasies free. Imagine cumming with your partner or what it feels like for your partner with you being the bottom. Experiment with as many positions as possible to find the best mutual pleasure for both of you.

Some prostrainers enjoy doing solo prostate play before sex, while others do not, preferring to be more sensitive. Some couples enjoy incorporating prostate play into their foreplay routine before transitioning to sex. Experiment away!

Finally, let's discuss bottoming. If you do explore getting pegged, **go slow and use a depth limiter** (which looks like an extended cock ring) to make sure the dildo does not penetrate you too far. The gear you choose is also important. Choose a harness that's comfortable, won't scratch either of you, and stays securely in place without constant adjustments.

Pegging can be fun with the right partner. It is recommended that you start with some light toy play first and teach your partner about your prostate zone before going right into the pegging phase. You can start with gloved fingers, plugs, and small toys before you go for a full-on harnessed pegging session. Explain the rhythm you prefer, how your P-Gasms forms, what to do to have a dry orgasm, where to touch you, etc. And don't be afraid to add a bit of role-playing to make it more fun. **Constant communication is essential!**

As for the "real thing", many straight males admit that as they become more proficient in anal play, they begin to fantasize about taking an actual cock. Based on conversations, many men have told me there is nothing that replaces the feeling of a raw cock in the ass. Of course, there are varying opinions on this topic; to follow are a few anecdotal takes.

"My first anal orgasms happened at a party. I was getting fucked, and I played with myself during sex. I came so fast and thought it was over, but he kept pounding my ass. It hurt, but I decided to wait for him to finish. In a few minutes, something wonderful happened. My body changed from mild pain to pleasure. I started to feel intense pressure building below my scrotum. The pleasure grew and grew. The harder he went, the more waves of anal orgasms I had. As he came, I came too, and ended up squirting for the first time in my life. I learned that ejaculating first helps me achieve anal orgasms. I also learned that only a real cock makes me cum. Toys do not work."—Ricken H.

"I'm straight, been married for 20 years. I adore my wife. About three years ago, I got into prostate play, which led me to be curious about what a real penis would feel like. With permission, my wife let me seek it out. I was fucked three times. And I learned that nothing in my toy chest compares to the real thing. When you are getting fucked, you can let go of doing and just feel the pleasure better. Plus the intimate and forbidden pleasure for me is such a turn-on. I cannot recreate this with toys or machines. But be warned! You may want it over and over again, unable to stop seeking it. For me, it is starting to become the only thing that excites me now. Be careful of what you wish for if you seek out real dicks." —August F.

"Personally, toys are better for me because you are pin-pointing the prostate area that you love to stimulate. Unlike when you're getting fucked, you lose that control. You do get to relax and enjoy some sensations, but the top is not always trying to focus on what feels good for you. A good top, which is rare, will want to figure out what feels good for you. But if their cock is not the right size and angle, forget feeling anything! Plus, most guys can't last long. It takes me a good while to awaken my prostate and get my anal orgasms going. Don't get me wrong, I like being a bottom, but it is rarely as good as the fantasy that's living in my head. And then there are STDs you need to worry about. I think this is overrated." -—Jose S.

"Being gay, I've had many cocks and toys in my ass. Almost always, it feels way better to have a real dick hitting the prostate. Even if you subtract the emotional and attraction part of sex, cock just hits better. And a partner can sense the spots that feel good, and you can guide him to the sweet spots. The best part is the throbbing, hot feeling. No toy can do this! When you get close to having an anal orgasm, you can just melt and get pounded into waves of pleasure. Machines and toys are super fun, but have no real attributes, and they cannot adjust to hit the right spots, or stop if it hurts you. Real cocks are also better because when he cums inside you, there is nothing else like this feeling: the heat, contact, and union. The pulsating and warm ooze always makes me have an instant anal orgasm." —Jesse T.

"I've fantasized about being fucked, but I'm not attracted to men, not even a cock. I think it's just the *idea* of being fucked by another guy that arouses me. I guess you can say it is my brain and not my hole that craves getting fucked. Haven't done it yet. Although at this point, I'd probably consider myself heteroflexible and not straight anymore since I have these thoughts. Getting more into prostate orgasms made me realize that gender and sexual identity blur quickly. I sometimes watch gay anal and trans porn, and I imagine myself being the bottom. Might happen eventually, but I doubt it." —Timothy B.

For any kind of penetrative sex, communication, STI test-ing, and plenty of lube are important. Discovering the right pleasure spots with a partner can lead to climaxes that solo play can't match. Remember, properly planned anal sex does not hurt. Take time to explore and understand what you like, and don't like, so you can find out what works best. Even if a prostate orgasm escapes you, chances are you'll have some type of intense mutual pleasure along the way. It may take some experimenting to figure it out. So go slow and enjoy all the pleasure this experience has to offer.

CHAPTER 23

EROTIC HYPNOSIS AKA "HYPNOFETISHISM"

Overview

- Discover how erotic hypnosis can enhance pleasure and deepen arousal.
- Cue Laszlo or Nadja's voice in a Staten Island office whispering, "You will have an anal orgasm"

Erotic hypnosis can tease, tantalize, and take your kinks to new levels of pleasure. It can also encourage deep states of sexual arousal. By default, many of us let the body lead the mind. But you can use hypnosis as a tool to guide the mind, allowing the body to follow as its servant.

As emphasized throughout this book, the key is relaxation, breathing, and focus. Hypnosis helps to downregulate your body by using relaxation and breathing techniques. A hypnotist's job is to guide you into a trance-like state using verbal instruction (inductions, triggers, and suggestions). Best of all, hypnosis can be used for reaching a hands-free orgasm.

In a deep state of hypnosis, transformations can occur in the mind and body. Relaxation washes over the body, while conscious awareness of the past and present world gently fades into the background. This altered state of consciousness focuses the subject's attention on the speaker, making them more open to suggestions. I personally don't believe a hypnotherapist can brainwash you into doing something against your will. To me, hypnosis is more like entertainment—a kind of 3D mental porn that taps into your imagination and amplifies your experience. It can be a tool that, when used intentionally, helps you unlock new levels of arousal.

Some hypnosis-themed content blurs the line of consent, especially if it portrays mind control, coercion, or manipulation. Always ensure consent, safety, and control. Hypnosis should enhance pleasure, not override free will.

Try hypnosis for more pleasure during anal sessions. When you follow a speaker's instructions, the guided journey shifts your focus entirely toward pleasure. It puts your mind in a suspended state, making orgasms happen more easily. It can also bring out things that might otherwise stay hidden and lower your inhibitions. A hypno-orgasm can be a fun and wild experience if you're willing to temporarily give up control.

I highly recommend hiring a professional hypnotist to create custom hypnosis files tailored to your needs. The cost for an audio file typically ranges from $100 to $300 (USD). Check out **Thervo**, a website that matches you with a hypnotist depending on your location. Or, **Psychology Today** offers a list of hypnotists in your local area. You can also find an expert by googling, word of mouth, or searching kink forums. Always verify each hypnotist's credentials to avoid being scammed or abused.

Honorable Mention: Search the web for the following terms: **JOI, HypnoTube, KinkyShibby.** There is a video online called "Anal6" with really good hypnosis and triggers. **Reddit (r/EroticHypnosis, r/SissyHypno)** and **thehypnocollective.com** also are places to find free files. But don't expect to find many good ones for free. High-quality hypnosis files focused on anal play and hands-free orgasms will likely need to be purchased at warpmymind.com, clips4sale.com, or erotic-hypnosis.com.

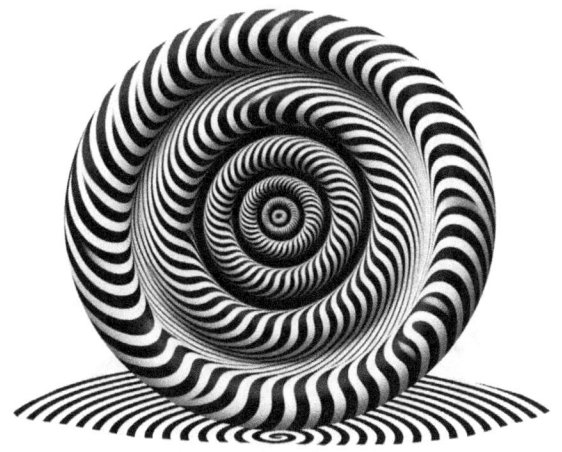

Hypno helps dissolve the resistance in your mind like a sugar cube in hot coffee.

CHAPTER 24

EQUIPMENT IS EVERYTHING

Overview

- There's a wide range of sex toys and accessories, from dildos and electric or app-controlled devices to furniture and more.
- Experiment with accessories and equipment designed to enhance arousal and pleasure.
- Use trial and error to find the perfect toy for your needs and experience level.
- Everything but the kitchen sink—minus that new erotic looking faucet you just bought.

⚠ Improper use of adult equipment can result in serious injury or harm. Always follow the manufacturer's guidelines, safety instructions, and operational procedures before use. Ensure that all safety features are in place and functioning properly. Failure to do so can lead to personal injury, damage to the machine, or other hazardous conditions. Be sure to use caution and act responsibly with your sex equipment.

Unless you are strictly doing mental orgasms, you're going to need the right tackle when playing with your ass. Fortunately, we are living in a golden age of prostate toys and Amazon is the Harbor Freight of sex tools! Sales of sex toys have been surging over recent years. And the consumer driver for this trend has been mostly straight cis men. Be warned though . . . collecting sex toys can be an addictive and expensive hobby. You were warned!

Whatever you choose to buy, **always use a toy with a base that prevents it from slipping too far inside you**. Again, no one wants to end up in the ER at 11 PM with a nurse digging her hands into your sphincter to retrieve a lost toy. And don't tear your ass! Be careful when experimenting with toys. Often they do not come with warning stickers or manuals!

My top recommended picks that are popular and effective*:

- Topped Toys – Hilt
- Bad Dragon – Echo the Snow Strider®, Sleipnir, Crackers®
- Aneros – Eupho, Syn Trident, MGX, Progasm, Vice
- Lelo – Billy, Bruno, Hugo, Loki Wave 2
- VixSkin – Mustang, Creations
- Uberrime – Splendid
- Lovense – Edge 1 & 2, Osci 2
- Nexus – Revo Stealth, Sparta
- njoy – Pfun Plug, Pure Plug, Pure Wand
- SquarePegToys – Charlie Horse, MegaMilkIt, Big Stick
- Avant – D3-4 or D11-12
- Tantus – Pspot, Prostate Play, Uberrime Astra
- WeVibe – Ditto, Vector

*Note: Some models may have updated versions with slight name and number variations. The versions listed do not imply they are the best or only ones to purchase.

Sex toys are like power tools—they might not be necessary for every job, but when you use them, they make everything faster, smoother, and way more exciting. Unfortunately, you start with one trusty drill, and suddenly you've got a whole shed full of gadgets you rarely use. That rotary tool seemed like a great idea at the time, but now you're just staring at it wondering, "Why did I think I needed this for my nightstand project?"

Whatever you decide on buying, it is important to find a toy with the right curve that matches your prostate. Make sure it has the correct angle and applies the right pressure to your sweet spot. Size is a factor to consider as well. If it's too small, it might not hit your spot effectively; too big and it's a painful no-go.

Dildos

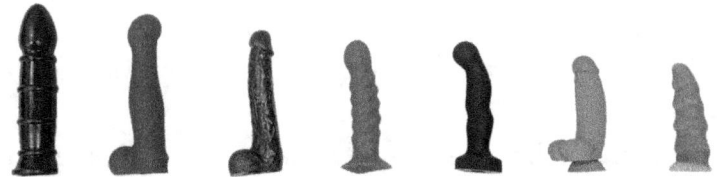

No one in the prostranal community has ever said, "This is the last dildo I will ever buy!" It's going to take a while to find the right one. And each one can work differently, depending on your mood and body. If you still don't have the right dildo in your toy collection, keep searching.

I've tried over 50 models and found, for me, the medium-soft, curved and smoother ones allow me to play longer, and have sessions without discomfort or soreness. But I also have a medium-hard toy that is scalloped and with ridges. When my sex machine is dialed up to 8 out of 10, it can bring a river of cum that my soft dildo cannot match. The only downside I've found with many grooved and textured hard dildos is that they start feeling uncomfortable after 10–20 minutes—kind of like driving on a road full of speed bumps. If you're going for textured dildo, a softer material is the way to go. But hey, maybe you like it rough and hard. You do you.

Dildos are typically made of one of these materials:

- Silicone
- PVC
- Stainless Steel
- Wood
- Jelly
- Ceramic
- Plastic (hard ABS)
- Glass
- Rubber
- Minerals (quartz, obsidian, malachite, amethyst, etc.)

Silicone is the most popular because it is (generally) nontoxic, nonporous, and not as hard as the others listed. Good-quality silicone is also more expensive because it's (typically) a high-quality material. There is nothing wrong with using the other types; just make sure the materials are nontoxic (phthalate or lead-free).

The other problem with going outside of silicone is that

some of the other materials are porous and difficult to sanitize (i.e., think sponge that can harbor bacteria). Remember that many of the cheaper Chinese knockoffs (silicone included) are not body-safe and toxic-free. **You need to be careful what you buy and stick in your ass!**

I recommend that you only buy quality platinum-cured silicone that is nonporous and hydrophobic. Stay away from mineral dildos as well. Some can be safe, but you never know exactly what you are getting when you buy online. Additionally, minerals can interact with the biological substrate in negative ways, causing allergic reactions and possible infections.

Whichever dildo you buy, consider the firmness and softness as major factors in reaching orgasm. Some prostrainers demand hard, kneading pressure. Others prefer a softer squeezing or rolling sensation on their prostate. And others need something in the middle. If you want the feeling that closely resembles a penis, use a dual-density dildo. It has a unique feel since it is a two-layer toy, and these tend to be the most comfortable for newbies.

> Everything's bigger in Texas, except your toy collection. Until 2008, Texas had an obscenity law making it a crime to own more than six dildos. Challenged and eventually overturned, it became famous for spotlighting the state's bizarre attempts to regulate personal pleasure.

Each dildo comes with a different "shore hardness". There is actually a scientific scale for measuring the hardness of different materials using classifications and number scales. They can be measured on a scale called a shore durometer. Fortunately, you don't need to use a calculator since most toy makers only list the toy as either soft, medium-soft, medium-hard, or hard.

But even with these descriptors, **the size of the toy heavily influences how the rectum reacts when forces are applied**. Know your anal physics and figure out your tolerance for thrust, pressure, etc. You need to choose the right size and silicone shore based on your preference. For example, a small soft dildo might be stubborn to insert and wiggle out too easily. And a large hard one might be more difficult to take, compared to a large soft one. Or, an XL might fit as a soft, but not as a medium shore. Some toy makers are now offering variations on firmness. Bad Dragon has the option for a soft shaft with a firm base, or medium shaft with firm base. There's lots to consider when it comes to silicone.

To achieve a prostate orgasm, you need to find a shape that effectively reaches and massages your prostate. I recommend a shape that grows thicker in the middle and has a nice rounded, wide head. Some like the feeling of fullness; others like it to snake around and bounce inside their hole. I recommend a flexible, softer and smooth material at first. The Tantus P-Spot is an excellent toy for beginners, especially for use on sex machines. You can get into the fantasy "ogre-unicorn-alien" dildos later on in your practice.

When using your dildo, play with the geometry. Rotate the toy to find the right feel and see if it feels better at different axis points. If you can angle it, curve the dildo upward toward your belly while practicing control by squeezing your muscles around it. Play with as many different positions as possible. **Aim the dildo toward the tailbone** and do a few reverse kegels. This straightens, shortens, and sensitizes the ass; and relaxes it in terms of width, letting the dildo pass through comfortably, and hopefully with pleasure. The sensitive areas on that front wall of the rectum will seek the head of the toy and do its best to find that delicious balance between discomfort and joyous friction.

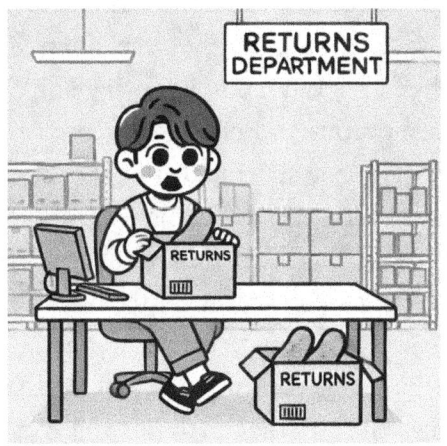

Toy selection is a trial-and-error process, and there is no guarantee of how it will feel once you start using it. Unfortunately, for obvious reasons, all sales are final—once you buy it, it's yours to keep!

The ideal proportions for me are 7-10 inches insertable in length, with a diameter thickness of around 1.70-2.25 inches. If your dildo is too long, it will cause discomfort and hit too deep. You can use any size you choose, but it does not need to be very long. Remember, **the prostate is just a few inches inside you.** It really will come down to finding the right thickness, texture, and angle.

Some of my dildo pro tips:

- Before play, soak your dildo in warm water, or run it in the microwave for a few seconds. This will make it feel much better. No one likes a cold dildo—especially in the winter. **CAUTION: Do not insert anything that is hot and could burn you!**
- Wash your silicone toys in the dishwasher (not on the hot, dry setting) and only wash silicone dildos in a dishwasher. I recommend only using silicone dildos, as others are porous and not as hygienic.
- If you are using a sex machine (which I recommend!) many dildos do not come with a Vac-U-Lock pre-drilled hole; they only have a suction pad or proprietary adapters. You will need to make this hole in your dildo, and it is easy to do with a drill if you have DIY experience. Mounting on a vise or fixed clamp, get a spade drill bit (that matches the rod size) and center the drilling about 2" deep directly in the center. Just be careful not to drill through the sides and tear it open. Use precision—or don't attempt this at all. If the hole is already pre-drilled (larger Vac-U-Lock pre-drilled hole), you can buy the Lovense or Hismith attachment bolts and just jam them in the base hole of your dildo. I recommend getting a spring attachment if you do.

Funny Side Note: The timeline and evolution of dildos has a humorous curve for most straight cis gender men. It goes something like this:

1. Man discovers his finger feels good in his butt.
2. Man asks partner to use finger.
3. Man uses vegetable, but realizes this is not sustainable, and now feels shame buying cucumbers, even if it is for his salad.
4. Man buys first non-phallic sex toy. Usually beaded looking or tapered.
5. Man needs bigger non-phallic toy and buys another in a different shape or style.
6. Man says, "I am never getting a penis-looking dildo because it will make me gay" and he'd be terribly embarrassed if someone were to find it.
7. Man buys first phallic dildo . . . and loves it.
8. Man buys black cock dildo so it doesn't show the brown stains from when he accidentally shits on it during prostate play.
9. Man buys many more dildos of different densities and sizes.
10. Man buys fantasy dildo with some knotty base that looks like an alien or Orc cock.
11. After many years, man finally finds a "Goldilocks" dildo that is just right. In his closet is a suitcase with well-worn sex toys that'll never be used again. Maybe only to superglue them all onto a mean neighbor's fence as a prank someday.
12. This man is me.

Aneros Toys

High Island Health (HIH) originally developed a medical device for prostate health, but unexpectedly, these prostate massagers gained recognition as pleasure devices. And that's sort of how Aneros was born.

Today, Aneros is one of the top prostate massage manufacturers in the world. And their popularity keeps growing more mainstream. These simple yet ergonomic toys provide a unique orgasmic experience compared to other prostate toys. It's like acupressure for the inside of your butt. They rhythmically and slowly rub and compress the prostate while also stimulating the anus, rectal walls, K-Spot, and perineum. These slow, rolling massages synchronize with your pelvic floor exercises.

Aneros toys create the perfect pleasure feedback loop through slow, delicate sensations. This stimulation triggers involuntary contractions, which, in turn, intensify the loop, building arousal, leading to orgasm. The more stimulation, the stronger the orgasms. The more orgasms, the greater their intensity and frequency. This continuous cycle is what makes them so effective.

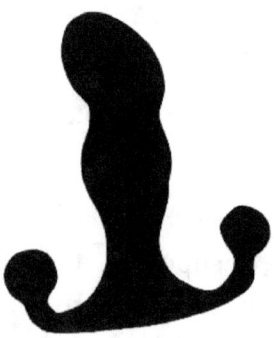

Aneros toys are like driving a manual stick shift—sure, it takes a little more practice and finesse, but once you master it, the control and precision are incredibly satisfying. Unlike other sex toys that might feel like driving an automatic, Aneros toys make you an active participant, fully engaged in every curve and shift along the way.

You insert it, start your kegels, and let it take off down the road to orgasm. This allows you to focus on the pleasure. I was skeptical until I purchased one. However, after a somewhat steep learning curve, I became a believer. And I've discovered that Aneros has a cult following with forums online. If you choose to join one of them, this support community will gladly show you the way.

The Aneros toy is designed to be constantly moving, regardless of how relaxed or tight you are. I recommend the Progasm and Maximus for a stuffed feeling of fullness. However, there is a downside to this: It doesn't move around as much and feels a little bit big and snug for some users. On the flip side, the Helix and Eupho toys move around a lot more—they crawl around, tickling the best spots inside your ass. I also love this feeling. That is why I bought a Progasm (Trident) and a Eupho (Syn). Keep in mind when purchasing, there are different series. The Aneros primarily uses two types of materials: the Trident series is made of hard thermoplastic, while the Syn series is made of soft silicone. I also recommend their vibrating models—they're great to have inserted during sex with a partner.

For those who have the time, set aside at least 1-2 hours when you start a session with an Aneros toy. **Focus on the sensation you are receiving, and let the orgasmic waves build slowly.** You can do kegels and reverse kegels, rock back and forth with a pillow, or just stay still and do nothing. It comes down to controlling the pelvic-floor muscles and nerve network surrounding the prostate, while slowly creating long-period waves of pleasure and circular orgasms.

Focus on the pleasurable sensations with your mind's eye, then slowly introduce a P-Muscle contraction, and hold it. Try an A-Muscle contraction. Play with variations (waves, pulsing, long holds, etc.). Flex these muscles as slowly as you can. The pleasure rises as you increase the intensity and "bite down" on it with your sphincter. Keep repeating it as slowly as possible making sure you relax your body's muscles. I strongly encourage you to revisit the breathwork, pelvic floor, and A-less exercises from the previous chapters while using an Aneros toy. And Mindgasm works great with an Aneros toy, too!

The key to using an Aneros is finding the perfect balance between tension and relaxation. You will notice stronger toy movement once your involuntary contractions form—it will move on its own. Once you learn to isolate the right muscles, it will feel like you are effortlessly rolling and thrusting your toy along the landing pad of your prostate gland. Always make sure you look at the shape of your toy, and have it inserted the correct way inside you (the curve facing your navel).

Again, this type of play is not a sprint. Much like a marathon, it requires patience. Create the right setting in the room. Really get into the moment and put everything else on hold. Most users lack patience, but making time for this toy truly pays off.

If you can fully get into the right headspace, relax and enjoy the sensations, your body will take over and do the rest. For instance, I like to rest with it inside me for an hour or so when I go to sleep; and then be woken up by contractions and orgasms as I drift between awake and dream states, and enjoy the slow, strong, and endless orgasms. Use a body-safe, oil-based lube if you decide to do this. This helps protect your anal walls from chaffing. Many prefer the brand Elbow Grease, or good old-fashioned coconut oil.

The Aneros is more like a tantric toy. Avoid pushing on it, shaking or externally vibrating it, or bouncing on it. You do not need to touch it once it is inserted, unless you are adjusting it. If you are lucky, you might instantly feel P-Waves and dry orgasms in seconds. Some advanced prostrainers have experienced involuntary contractions and even Super-Os within minutes of their first time using it.

Make sure you begin breathing in and out, with long, slow rhythms when you start using it. Once you get a good rhythm going, do small, anal contractions as you are breathing. Inhale and contract your anus. And when you exhale, release the anal contraction. Keep doing this with your breathing over and over, slowly making your breathing deeper and your contractions harder. **Breath is everything with this toy!** Revisit the earlier chapters on breathwork and pelvic floor exercises while experimenting with your Aneros.

Your Aneros will also work better when you play with the various positions. To get started, I prefer to be on my back lying down with my legs lightly spread, relaxing with some music or Mindgasm. I also enjoyed sitting down at my desk and having it inside while I wrote portions of this book. Also while driving (safely). In all instances, I like to slightly rock back and forth in my seat.

I recommend trying it while lying on your side too. You can rock back and forth in this position or make your body slither like a snake in the bed. This can create the wave patterns that bring the most pleasure. Standing works as well. Put your hands on your head and slightly bend back and forth. Or play with doggy style, where you grab a pillow and do a slight rising and falling of your abdomen. Incorporate your kegel exercises in any position when using your Aneros.

You can even try a short 10-20 minute online Yin yoga class while using one.

> **Pro Tip:** There are many ways to use an Aneros. For example: do a reverse kegel (P-Muscle), but only lightly push out and hold. Keep it constantly pushing out, and don't worry if you use a little bit of your A-Muscle as well here. Do this kegel ever so light while imagining the muscle in your perineum pushing out. Focus on the feeling and maintain your breathing. If you don't feel anything, leave it in for a while longer. Do this lying on your side; or your back with your legs up against a wall.

E-stim

If an Aneros sounds difficult, imagine sending volts of electricity to your most sensitive parts in order to orgasm . . .

E-stim uses electrical currents to target muscles and nerves, stimulating your nervous system. Wires from the e-stim device are attached to electrode sticky pads, rubber loops, and even butt plugs. Steady streams of electrical pulses are delivered through these wires from the e-stim unit. The units are small enough to fit in your hand, though some are larger. Like a DJ, you play with all the buttons and settings to find the right mix of pleasure. The pulses of electricity make the muscles stimulated and aroused. By causing repeated muscle contractions, both penile and anal orgasms can be achieved.

You can buy e-stim anal toys online that are geared for prostate play. I prefer the steel butt plugs over the silicone ones. Of course, e-stim has many complexities and challenges. **It takes time to master, and e-stim is more difficult to excel in than most toys.** Your power box needs to have enough juice to stimulate and deliver the correct type of waveform. You need a special type of electrode that can be placed near or close to your prostate. It is different for everyone. Some enjoy placing the electrode pad on various areas: the perineum, the penis glands or shaft, or the thighs.

Expect the occasional jolt of pain or burning as you figure out these configurations through trial and error. Eventually, you will get interesting sensations and experience a simultaneous tingling in your penis, prostate, anus, and perineum.

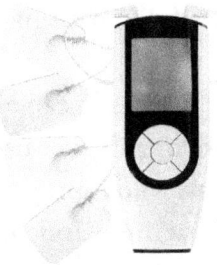

I recommend putting one pad on the perineum, positioned high, low, or in the middle; put one on the underside of the penis head gland. Also place one on the base of the shaft. Finally, if you do not buy an electrode plug, place a pad nearer to the anus to reach the prostate, but not directly on the hole. You can also place pads on the back of the knees, the lower back, and even the inside ankle.

Some have found that using an Aneros while doing e-stim can greatly enhance the experience and bring Super-Os. For added fun, use e-stim with a sex machine for heightened pleasure. Get creative. You will have to search and dig deep to learn about e-stim orgasms. Many online forums exist, and it is its own world.

But be warned—using e-stim can cause temporary numbness. It is commonly used in pain management to modulate nerve activity and reduce sensitivity.

> **Pro Tip**: Try the 64X Pro-Shocker Vibrating and E-stim Prostate Plug if you want a fun, electrifying experience. It has several unique modes (milk, squeeze, torment, etc.) made specifically for orgasm amplification.

! **WARNING**: E-stim can be dangerous. It can burn your body if you are not careful. It can also numb your pleasure zones if used for too long. **Never use it near your heart. And never allow a woman who is pregnant to use it. Follow the manufacturer's instructions and consult with a doctor before you use e-stim.**

njoy Pure Wand

This toy looks simple, but it can be complicated, since there are many ways to use it. Nevertheless, it's a heavy and steady toy that can get the orgasms flowing. I recommend you ease into things, especially if you are using the Pure Wand for the first time. You need to work your way up to some faster thrusting and deeper penetration. Avoid tearing yourself and go slow.

You might be used to softer and bendier toys that are more forgiving. This is not one of those—It's a heavy-duty toy!

When you get one, run it under warm water (not hot) before insertion. It retains heat well. Start by gently pressing the lubed ball into your lubed anal opening and carefully exerting some pressure. You decide which end to use. The smaller 1-inch ball is better to start with, especially if you're new to anal play. The handle of the wand has a curve to it; so use a gentle touch and feel your way deeper.

After entering the anal opening, feel for the inner wall of the rectum, and find a cold sensation in that spot. Spend some time here exploring the seminal vesicle area. It can be quite pleasurable. **The key is finding the right depth.** Use gentle poking motions, easing a bit more of the tip each time you poke. Thrusting it in and out very fast and at different depths is very dangerous.

If you are not used to intense prostate stimulation, it can feel like a shock the first time. The Wand initially creates a strange sensation, but it will soon wash over to a pleasurable one. There is no need to grind it hard and deep into your prostate as soon as you make contact. Use a light touch until you can figure out how much pressure feels right. You'll eventually notice something wonderful happens when the rounded ball makes contact with your prostate. You will likely feel both aroused and as if you suddenly need to pee. As with most prostrainers, you will have to learn to pass through the "have to pee" stage to get to the anal orgasm.

The key for me is to pull the Wand upwards, so it puts pressure on the prostate, and presses up to the inner part of the perineum. This sandwiching of the two areas, along with the force of thrusting, quickly sends me into squirt mode.

The hardest part is that all the action strains my wrist, leaving it feeling like I have carpal tunnel afterward. If you have a partner, put them to work, and guide them as you explore. If you don't have a partner, switch hands, go two-handed, or take regular breaks.

I recommend trying the reverse insertion method. Many people have experienced their first prostate orgasm sometimes within a minute of using this technique. Start by lying on your side, in the fetal position. When you are comfortable, insert the small end of the Wand inside you. Keep the bigger ball running away from your lower spine. Instead of having the curve of the Wand hooking up along your tailbone and balls, or curving along your back, turn it the opposite way, so it looks like you a have a tail *(see image for reference)*. Reach around and pull it up and down, to locate your favorite spots. You can also flip it around the other way, so the large ball side runs along the curve of your spine. Experiment with a variety of angles and variations until you discover which one feels the best.

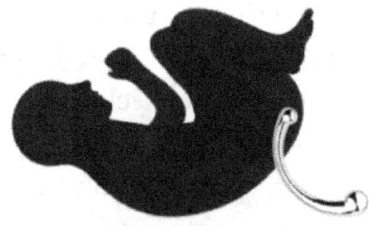

I call this the "Rock-a-Bye Baby" technique.

Keep pushing it in and out, all around, and explore. This will stimulate a much bigger prostate area and bring intensified pleasure sensations. **It is a great way to stimulate the prostate for those who struggle to find their anal pleasure zones**.

Also, take a shot at doing it without using your hands. Instead, keep it inside of you, and do rocking or snaking motions; and/or making slight movements with your hips, creating come-hither motions. If done correctly, you'll be able to ride the wand, just using your hips up and down. Switch it up and use the larger ball if you wish. Always incorporate your PAT Method and breathwork.

Another variation is lying flat on your back with the wand curving underneath, i.e., imagine a metal tail pointing down. You want to grind on it. Hold the big end in place while repeatedly grinding your hips down into the mattress. Use a pillow, a jock strap, or underwear to keep it in place.

Note: There are cheap knockoffs on the market. But beware: some of them can contain lead or other harmful materials. Always use caution when shopping for a wand.

"I lie on my back, legs spread far apart, putting the soles of my feet together, forming a triangle. I slowly pull the Wand back and forth over my prostate. After a few light orgasms, I gradually increase the speed and pressure until the Super-Os arrive. I stop when I'm out of fluid, dizzy, and too sensitive to go on." — Thad

Self-Massage Canes

A self-massage cane (like a Thera Cane®) is used to apply pressure to muscles. The unique design of this kinky candy cane lets you apply deep pressure to massage hard-to-reach areas of your body. It was developed by a chronic pain patient; but sure enough, the prostrainer community gave it a try, and devised a way to make the Cane a chronic pleasure device.

This amazingly simple-yet-effective device makes it easy to reach your prostate once you learn how to pinpoint the position and techniques. It is fairly inexpensive and simple to use.

Self-massage canes are made of plastic and not body-safe or toxic-free. Remember, anytime you are inserting something inside you, it should be made of body-safe materials. So use a condom if you do decide to play with one. And you might need to sand down the round part (using a light grit) since it can be rough. Any of the positions you choose need to be done carefully and with caution. Go slow and move slowly.

First, start on your knees with a pillow under each knee and straddle it like you would a pogo stick.

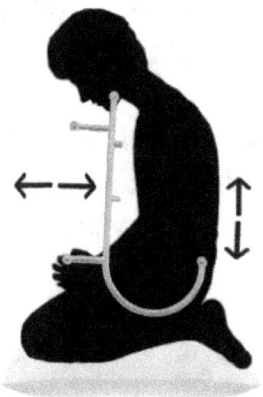

You can insert, and ride it up and down, or make a rocking motion back and forth ever so slightly. Less is more, especially when you are finding your pleasure spots.

I do not recommend the following riskier methods because of safety reasons. Some use the self-massage cane standing. Holding it with their hands, while others try rigging things, to figure out ways to have it glide along hands-free. They use anything elastic, such as a bungee cord to give it some play so it feels like it is moving on its own. If this all seems overly dangerous and complex, then just lie back on your bed and slowly try exploring yourself manually.

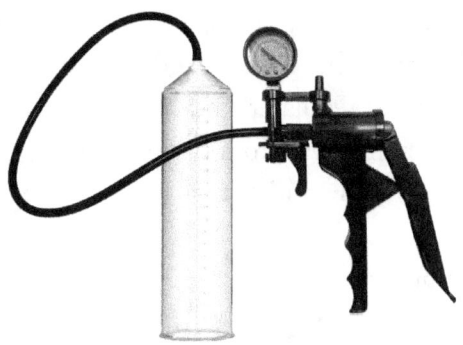

Penis Pumps

Remember the infamous scene in *Austin Powers* where the groovy spy is caught with a penis pump and adamantly denies ownership? "That's not mine, baby!" Sure, it was played for laughs, but it put penis pumps on the map as both a punchline and a curiosity. Jokes aside, penis pumps are real devices with serious prostate enhancement potential not just for humor, but for performance and satisfaction. Designed to increase blood flow and create firmer erections, they've become a valuable tool for sexual wellness. So, let's put the jokes aside (for now) and explore how they actually work.

A penis pump (vacuum device) gets your penis hard to sup-posedly increase length and girth. It can also be used during prostate play to help with prostate orgasms and open new pleasure pathways. Typically, a penis pump is made up of (1) a plastic or glass tube that fits over your penis, (2) a pump attached to the tube, and (3) a ring that fits around the base of the penis once it's erect to maintain your erection. I recommend the LeLuv Maxi Penis Pumps with a plastic ring. They are pricey, but in my opinion the experience is worth it!

Remember, penis pumps do not make your penis bigger permanently. And these devices are very dangerous when used incorrectly. **Discuss this with your doctor before using one!** Penis pumps are not regulated and could lead to serious injury. I recommend staying away from them or getting a penis pump prescribed by a doctor, and that is an FDA approved medical device.

If you try one, always pay attention to how your penis feels during the first few pumps. If something starts to hurt, immediately stop using it. These pumps can break the blood vessels in your penis and permanently affect the tissue, causing lifelong damage. **Only use a penis pump with a pressure gauge so you can monitor the pressure and keep it at a safe level.** Some users recommend that you never go past -10 mmHg and only use it once a day for less than 10 minutes (pressurized).

A penis pump coupled with a percussion gun or sex machine can squeeze your cock nicely, and help you feel the contractions during your kegels. This can speedily assist with rewiring and better understanding your pleasure paths.

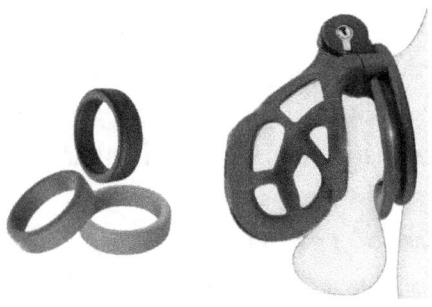

COCKS RINGS AND CHASITY CAGES

Let's talk about accessory equipment that enhances the anal play experience. Cock rings and chastity cages might sound like you would find them in a Medieval castle, but both are designed to unlock a whole new level of sensation and control during prostate play. Cock rings are the party-starters, keeping things firm, intense, and ready for an encore. Chastity cages, on the other hand, are the ultimate tease, turning restraint into the main event. These toys are not insertable, but they can complement anal play.

Cock Rings

Using a cock ring is like pressing the pause button before the final big scene in a movie— you're just holding on as long as possible before the climax comes!

A good ring increases the pressure in the pudendal region. This nerve provides sensation to the penis, scrotum, and anus.

When you wear a cock ring, it increases sensations during prostate play. It slows blood flow out of your erect penis, and can make erections harder and longer-lasting, as well. Cock rings make anal play more intense and raise arousal. Best of all, they delay orgasm, creating a more intense penile orgasm, P-Waves, and anal orgasms

Cock rings, also known as penis rings, tension rings, and constriction rings, liven up your sessions and come in all forms:

- Soft and stretchy rings are the most common and generally low priced. They are made of a soft material, often silicone. Easy to use and remove.
- Adjustable cock rings use lasso adjusters, Velcro, or other fasteners to fit your penis.
- Vibrating cock rings have a small vibrator attached. This might feel odd at first, and it will often force a penile orgasm before an anal orgasm.
- Solid cock rings are only for highly experienced users, since there is a danger of penis strangulation—especially with metal cock rings that fit poorly, get stuck, or are left on too long.

When used correctly, cock rings will not cause pain. If you want to wear a more complex cock ring setup (e.g., over your testicles), slide them in one ring at a time so they fit snugly, but are not uncomfortable.

Since cock rings restrict blood flow, **it is important not to wear one for longer than 20-30 minutes.** Allow around at least 60 minutes between uses. **A cock ring should fit well around the penis without causing pain or discomfort.** Do not go to asleep while using the ring. And do not use one in combination with drugs or alcohol. It could lead to potential injury and permanent damage.

Fortunately, there are safer options available. You can safely wear these two rings for more than 20 minutes without any harm. **FirmTech's MaxPR** and **Oxballs' Cocksling Air** are both excellent options that allow you to wear them longer than typical cock rings due to their stretchy, well-researched design. I love using them for sex, prostate play, or even solo sessions—they seriously boost pleasure.

Chasity Cages

These are the ultimate tool for sexual submission. They cage the penis under lock and key to prevent erection, self-pleasure, or any touching. And they are unlockable to only to you or your Dom.

Many find that chastity cages can be a useful tool in anal training for orgasms. Some say the cage forces you to ignore the front side so you focus exclusively on the back side. It requires you to resist an erection which will teach you to focus on your muscle groups, instead of your cock. Starving your erection can also change how you experience anal pleasure, and it can enhance your sensations.

For safety, a chastity cage should never hurt any part of your body. Make sure that you work up to wearing the cage for long periods. You have to find the right fit. Caging isn't for everyone. Depending on the user, cages can raise prostate sensitivity. To have some more fun, use a Hitachi-type vibrator (light setting) on your cage when playing with your prostate; that is, if you want to edge to orgasm. The vibration, especially with metal and plastic cages, can easily bring you close to a penile ejaculation. Even though we mostly focus on anal orgasms, sometimes you may just want to have a regular penis orgasm.

Remember that a cage is intended to keep your erection from growing. But many cages have a release, in case of an emergency, if your penis starts to outgrow its cage. Do not use a cage if it doesn't have this feature and remove it immediately if you feel any pain. Overall, **I do not recommend that you use a lock due to the risk of injury**.

> I once asked my firefighter friend to share one of his wildest stories, and he didn't disappoint. He told me about a late-night emergency call to a house party where a guy, decked out in leather, had a metal cock ring stuck—and was absolutely panicked. His groin had swollen so much that the ring needed to be cut off with a specialized tool. The moral of the story? Enjoy these accessories but always use them responsibly. Trust me, you don't want your wild night to end with a team of firefighters standing around you with a pair of bolt cutters!

Fingers

Last but not least . . . using a finger for prostate play is one of the most accessible and natural ways to explore prostate stimulation, whether you're new to it, or looking to deepen your experience. Fingers get honorable mention in this chapter because they offer a level of control and sensitivity that no toy can fully replicate. A finger makes a great starting point for discovering what feels good and how your body responds to touch. It's also an excellent way to connect with yourself or a partner on a more personal and intimate level.

This is the most readily, least expensive, safest and under-rated equipment available. Some prostrainers can create orgasms with just their fingers dancing on their prostate. There are many techniques to explore, from wagging to flicking. If you can experiment and find the right method, you might never need to use sex toys. Above everything, fingers are dis-crete—so there is no need to hide them under the bed, or in the closet like dildos and other sex toys.

Some suggestions for exploring your hole with one or more fingers:

- Trim your nails.
- Use a medical glove with lots of lube.
- Go very slow, do not force any movements.
- Find a comfortable position that works for your body type, e.g., sitting on a chair with your legs elevated. Resting against a wall. In your bed, lying on your side. Squatting on your knees.
- Use a thumb to tickle, wiggle, massage, or flick the prostate.

Don't forget that while fingers are fun, the hand and fingers fatigue easily. This might not provide right anal physics for anal orgasms.

If you can find a partner—one who is emotionally, eroti-cally, and physically connected—try having them finger you.

A partner can easily find and stimulate your prostate with a finger, especially if you communicate well with them. A partner's skilled fingers are definitely better than solo play.

For many, using a finger allows for greater feedback than external tools. You adjust your finger pressure and movements in real-time based on how it feels on your prostate. Best of all, a finger can give you the ultimate "five-finger discount" by getting you off without needing any fancy gadgets.

CHAPTER 25

THRUSTING, VIBRATING, ROTATING . . .

Overview

- Prostate massagers are popular, portable, and perfect for targeted stimulation.
- Not all vibrators give the same vibe, so choose wisely.
- Percussion guns deliver intense, heavy-duty stimulation.
- You'll never look at a reciprocating saw—or power tools—the same way again.

Prostate toy design has revolutionized the world of pleasure, offering tools that can take your experience to entirely new heights. Among the most exciting innovations are thrusting, vibrating, and rotating prostate massagers—each designed to unlock sensations you never knew existed. With a recent surge in popularity, the market is brimming with options, ranging from sleek and simple to high-tech and multifunctional. These toys aren't just about stimulation; they're about exploration, control, and discovering what really makes you tick. Whether you're new to prostate play or a seasoned explorer, these gadgets are worth checking out. The engineering and ingenuity are evolving faster than I keep up with these days.

Prostate Massagers

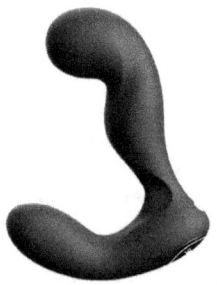

I am referring primarily to the electronic ones here. The ones that that look like joysticks or gear shifters. These stumpy devices come with many types of vibrating patterns, rotating heads, e-stim, inflatable, tapping functions, variable speeds, LED lights. They even come with remote controls and apps for your phone.

At the low end, the starting price is around $30 (USD), and they can go up to $200 (USD) and beyond. The cheaper online ones are generally okay but be cautious and check for the chemicals and materials used to make some of them before you buy. Most are not tested in US labs for quality control. Many low-end ones do have a variety of vibrating, pulsating, escalating actions that you can play with to hit the right spot. Unfortunately, these massagers can be loud and usually have short battery life. I recommend that you avoid the models with a removable bullet vibe, and get the USB-charging ones, since they are stronger and last longer.

Whatever model you buy, make sure it has a rounded end and flared base, so it doesn't disappear into your abyss. I prefer the massagers that hit/hug the perineum and thrust, or do the come-hither motion. I also enjoy the ones that are app based, offering varied and customizable vibration patterns. Try one with an attached cock ring as well. No matter your preference, they're fun as the main event or as a warm-up—perfect for rocking back and forth while browsing the internet before a sex machine session. The pulsing of vibrations and thrusts offers a comforting rhythm for anal orgasms. And this can lead to seriously intense orgasms.

My top picks:

- Lovense – Edge 2 or 3
- Lelo – Hugo and Loki Wave
- SVAKOM – Iker Neo
- Aneros – Vibrating Helix Syn V
- Nexus – Revo 2
- PALOQUETH – 2-in-1 Anal Vibrator (nicely taps your prostate)
- CHEVEN – Wiggle Motion (gives an enjoyable come-hither feeling)
- Utimi – Inflatable Anal Plug (fun and unique)

The only drawback I've noticed is battery life with some. Most last around 30-50 minutes. Be sure to check the device's runtime before purchasing, and keep in mind that battery performance may diminish over time, depending on the quality of the battery. Planning ahead can save you from a mid-session power outage—which is the ultimate *bummer*!

> The art of using prostate massagers lies in the fine balance of letting go and holding on.

Vibrators

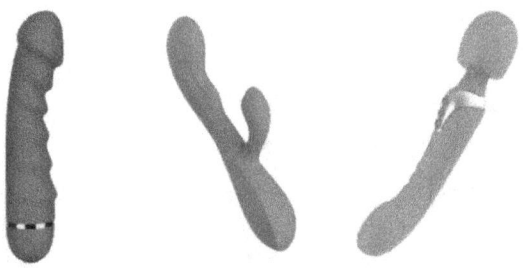

Many people think that vibrators are only for cis women and strictly designed for vaginas. But as you have already learned, both genders can have similar orgasms. More importantly, everyone has nerve endings and erogenous zones that respond to vibrating stimulation.

But vibration isn't for everyone. Many prostrainers prefer friction (thrust) over vibration. Some seasoned-prostate veterans believe vibrators are counterproductive to achieving anal orgasms, since they can desensitize and numb your prostate. Some disagree and love the sensation of a toy humming steadily in their ass, bringing them to climax.

As you've probably noticed in prostate play, everyone and everything is different. For some, prostate vibrators help massage the prostate more effectively and are a good entry point if pounding your prostate is uncomfortable. **Vibration adds**

stimulation to the prostate, potentially helping those with less sensitive prostates reach orgasm where other stimulation would not work.

Vibration stimulates both surface-level and deep nerves causing a unique pleasure sensation. The prostate-focused vibrators can provide much quicker motions and waves of stimulation, depending on your nerval structure. The key with vibrators is to find one that creates sparks of pleasure across your urogenital system. The best way to choose is to go to a sex shop and test out several brands. Do this by locating the small hollow just below your neckline, known as the "chest notch." Place the vibrator tip there. You'll typically experience three intensity levels: Level 1 stays localized to the point of contact; Level 2 spreads outward, reaching your chin and belly button; Level 3 radiates through your entire body, from head to toe. Each level can work. It depends on what you prefer.

I suggest you avoid "buzzy" vibrators. They tend to sound high-pitched and have low-wave intensity. This weaker vibration stays at the surface level and is not very satisfying. You'll most likely want the "rumbly" and "thumpy" vibrator that penetrates deeper into the body and spreads out, causing waves. Look for ones that give it all: pleasurable buzzing, deep thrumming, tickling or pulsing sensations. Hitachi, Nu Sensuelle, Lelo, We-Vibe and Lovense (Domi 2) have a rumbly/thumpy quality in their devices. Also, try using any vibrator at lower speed and power settings, especially when you start a session. Otherwise you might overpower and numb the nerves that give you pleasure.

Vibrators also work well when you are using another anal toy. Put it on your penis or perineum to build up your orgasm. Use a cock ring and attach it to your penis. Place the vibrator on your nipples, etc. Get creative. Just don't put it in your mouth, or you might have to make an emergency visit to the dentist.

Pro Tip: Some of the high-quality vibrating prostate toys are great to practice using the PAT Method. Find a vibration pattern that you can practice your kegels with. Incorporate with wave movements and pulsating holds during your pelvic floor contractions (e.g., PAT Method) to sync with the vibrations. For this, the **Lovense Osci** is the best option, since it has unlimited patterns that you can create; and it can sync with music and sounds.

Percussion Guns

These instruments have recently become a popular device for drilling the prostate. Many of these massage guns have a variety of weights, sizes, intensity, noise levels, battery life, and price points. The best ones use percussive therapy (rapid up and down motions with deep, rumbly vibrations). Avoid the ones that only vibrate and do not micro-thrust. These are just glorified vibrators that don't really "prostquake" you to orgasm. Find one with a very low setting to start but also has a powerful high setting. Many cheaper, inferior ones "jam up" when you clench too hard. Avoid these!

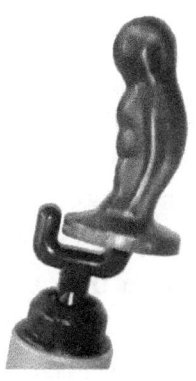

Placing a toy on the percussion gun can induce powerful full-body orgasms (both anal and penile). I've found the best method is to use the two-prong, fork attachment. Attach a smaller P-spot (curved) dildo to one end. You might need to drill a hole into it to fit. Use a fast-drying glue or epoxy to keep it in place. When you're ready to ride, let the open prong massage between your balls and anus. Start on the lowest setting and let the percussion massager do its magic. Relax, close your eyes, and ride the toy a little. Watch porn or do Mindgasm exercises. Then begin your kegel exercises. Try to maintain low-intensity kegels at first. Also, let your penis hang slightly so it is free and bouncing a bit. The vibrations can quickly bring an ejaculatory orgasm. It can get loud, so the best way to keep the sound down is to wrap the gun in a pillow. I use a knee wrap bandage to keep it in place. You can also use a belt. Once you get it snug, put two pillows on the side of it as you giddy-up like a cowboy, mounting it like a saddle. For extra comfort, put pillows under your knees so you can get the most angles and bounce.

My own experiences have been incredible! I have the

most intense anal and penile orgasms since the gun I use is heavy-duty and rumbles like a jackhammer. When the fork is applied to my perineum, I experience an intense tingling from inside my belly button. It is as though an electrical connection is established between the navel, balls, and tip of the penis. The feeling begins as a subtle tingle, then intensifies into a gripping wave that lasts for 10-15 minutes.

The anal contractions become so strong, and my penis repeatedly contracts and changes all directions from the spasms. After several anal orgasms, I usually end up squirting steady streams of prostatic fluid, followed by ropes of cum. Even though these orgasms are immediately satisfying, they are so addictive that I am wanting more anal and penile play later that day. The refractory period is shorter for me with these types of orgasms.

Percussion guns can also serve as a secondary stimulation tool, used simultaneously with a dildo, njoy Pure Wand, or sex machine. For example, using your gun for a perineum massage, or with a masturbator sleeve attachment or direct cock play can enhance pleasure. Also, you can break the rules and use your Aneros or other toy inserted with the gun on its lowest setting; place the foamy ball attachment on the tab or base of your butt toy, applying light to medium pressure on it; use pillows to stabilize the gun and hold it in place while you pinpoint the right spot.

If you don't consider yourself to be DIY-inclined, there are vendors online that manufacture dildos designed to be attached to a massage gun. Many sellers on **Etsy** and **Amazon** make percussion gun adapters, e.g., 3D-printed Vac-U-Lock adapters, silicone dildos, and more.

If you are struggling with these heavy-duty toys at first, try stroking your cock while riding one of them first, and having it turned off. When you reach a Level 6 arousal, power up the gun and focus on the sensations. Look for those tickling buzzes everywhere. Pump your hips to find the right rhythm and vibration. Only level up the power on the massager if you wish, but I recommend staying on a safe low to moderate setting. That should be enough to push you over the edge.

! WARNING: Many percussion devices are sold as pseudo-medical devices and are not intended for sexual purposes. Use at your own risk. Speak with your doctor before experimenting.

CHAPTER 26

SEX MACHINES

Overview

- Sex machines take hands-free pleasure to the next level with precision, power, and endless stamina.
- Master the best techniques and positions to maximize pleasure and effectiveness.
- James Brown said it best in "Get Up (I Feel Like Being a) Sex Machine" . . .

! Improper use of these machines can result in serious injury. Always follow the manufacturer's guidelines, safety instructions, and operational procedures while in use. Ensure that all safety features are in place and functioning properly. Failure to do so can lead to personal injury, damage to the machine, or other hazardous conditions. Be sure to use caution and operate responsibly.

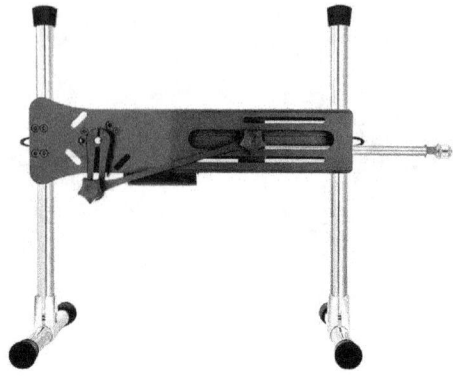

If you take your sexual pleasure seriously, then you are not likely to find anything more dedicated to making you have anal orgasms than a sex machine. Also known as "fuck machines", these powerful devices will provide multiple orgasms without the need for you to do anything—you just lie back and surrender to the endless strokes of pleasure. But buy a good one! You do not want to order one that stalls out when you start clenching or breaks after a few sessions. You get what you pay for. In my opinion, Hismith and Lovense set the gold standard for best price, customer support, and quality craftsmanship. Many cheap knockoffs do not have enough power and stop thrusting if you clench too hard. They also can be loud and leave almost no functionality for adjusting your settings. The other high-end expensive ones ($1,000+ USD) out there are always an option if you want to bravely splurge.

For example, I had a power supply issue and Hismith sent me a replacement part at their expense. Many of the cheaper and high-end models have a variety of issues and might not provide customer support. So take that into account. And many Hismith owners have machines that have lasted 10+ years. If you do get one, just make sure you grease the bearings and rod mount areas every year as part of your maintenance routine. And do not hit the power box (speed controller) and plug in leads hard because they are a bit delicate. I also recommend that you are careful with the wire leading out of the power box, since it tends to pull out from the box and strip easily.

When you first open the sex machine box, you might find yourself staring at it in wonder and confusion. Many people just shake their heads and think, *Where am I supposed to hide this fucking thing?*

The most important step when experimenting for the first time is figuring out the best angle and position to ram your ass. **Take time to play with this machine and go slow.** Do not expect to go straight into prostate play until you sort this out. Think about your anal physics here. Once you find the right position/angle for the machine, mark it with a piece of tape, or a Sharpie, so you can reset it when you change the angles or store it. The best position is the one where you can stay most comfortable (no cramping or effort) for as long as possible.

Alternate angles to find your P-Spot. The best angle creates a feeling like the dildo is scraping the roof of your rectum, especially when it gets right under the base of the cock, and you start to feel it generate warm tingles in the belly. Focus on this area, move around, and push down hard to intensify the involuntary contractions.

Additionally, it works best when the angle makes it feel like the dildo thrusts are pushing and putting pressure on your perineum. Find this sweet spot. In addition, clench your stomach area with one hard kegel, while simultaneously pushing out (a reverse kegel). I usually want the head of the dildo to barely exit so it almost pops and flicks the ring of my hole, stretching and sending more waves along the nerves of the canal.

> Remember this: The arm of the machine is the engine; your ass is the steering wheel. Move in the direction of pleasure.

Depth and speed vary for everyone. I generally prefer shallower strokes, but sometimes I will reset it to longer, deeper strokes. I also control how much my hole swallows up the toy. When I am getting close to orgasm, I shift my hips down and take every inch. As for speed, I always start slow. But toward the end of my session, that machine is near full speed.

Some ideas and variations:

- Use a gym weight bench. Play with the angles. Experiment with lying face down or lying face up.
- Use a chair. Put it against a wall. Hang your ass to the edge of the chair, prop your legs up on the wall, and have the machine angled up. Or sitting backward in a chair while on your computer.
- Flat on your back with knees to chest, widen and squeeze knees together to experiment with pressures on the prostate.
- Use a wedge pillow or stack several pillows under your chest for doggy style. Rub your cock while getting hammered and use a wand massager on your perineum.
- On your side works well; especially if you have your

cock squeezed between your thighs or flipped back (i.e., you can rub your cock with your thighs and do some fun ballooning).

- On your back, propped up with pillows under the upper back and head. Place legs in the air or bent for a spider pose.
- A sex swing or looping waist harness is great for finding the right angles and being able to really relax your body.
- Modify a chair (cut a hole in it) so the machine can pound you while you watch porn on your computer. Or, try the "bar stool anal" position. Hang your ass just off the edge of a bar stool and place a sex machine underneath you. Sit at your desk or bar, watching your favorite porn, or reading erotic fiction. Comfortably sit back and let your ass get pounded until you cum.
- Attach a cock ring to the dildo. Use a vibrating anal bead wand, or something similar, and put it through the cock ring so the base is hitting the perineum, and the tips are pressed on the testes. Or, you can also strap a vibrating toy to your dildo (i.e., I use my Hitachi wand with the penis massager and put it on the dildo so it vibrates it while I am receiving the thrusts.)
- Buy the Double Penetration Function Expander attachment and put two dildos on each end. Choose a shorter dildo for the top, so you can have it hang low and hit your perineum, while the bottom dildo is inserted inside you. If the top one doesn't hang down, try using a cock ring around both dildos at the base, so the top one creates friction on your scrotum, cock, and perineum. Turn it on and get a double whammy

of thrusting pleasure!

- If you don't get the aforementioned attachment, you can still use cock rings (or a penis sleeve) and attach another dildo on top of your prostate dildo. This way you can rub an extra dildo together with your penis as one dildo rams your ass and the other glides across your shaft.

! **SAFETY ALERT**: A fuck machine can really fuck you up! Never turn it on when the setting is on high and a toy is inside of you. Always keep the power off switch nearby. Do not plug it in near water; or daisy chain the connection creating an electrical or fire hazard. Consult with your doctor before buying one. Lastly, remember the golden rule: **Using a sex machine should be pain free and feel good. Do not continue using it if it hurts!**

The ultimate key is to just get used to letting the machine keep going and fucking you. It can help to fantasize about its relentlessness—that it will not stop until you cum. Or think about your partner, or a stranger fucking you hard. Let this submissive state take over and enjoy the endless thrusting.

Sex machines are wonderful because they will usually make you squirt, since your bladder is getting worked alongside your prostate. If this scares you, pee before a session, or go into your session slightly dehydrated. But if you do squirt, you can use towels, puppy pads, or a condom to capture your mess. The pushing sensations (i.e., peeing or pooing) can become powerful and feel uncomfortable; but just let it happen while you breathe and relax. This is when the deep powerful orgasms follow. **Always remember to stop if you feel pain!**

> **Pro Tip 1:** Use a vibrating wand (or equivalent) and use a TPE Male Humming Bird Attachment attached to your dildo. As the sex machine thrusts, you will get extra stimulation from the vibrations to your perineum, scrotum, and even penis base. It is better to use a longer dildo so you can avoid the attachment from hitting your sphincter. Or use a vibrating cock ring and attach it to the base of the dildo so you get that extra vibration during thrusting. Hismith makes dildos that have internal vibrators built in. It worth trying if you like both the feeling of vibration and thrusting at the same time.

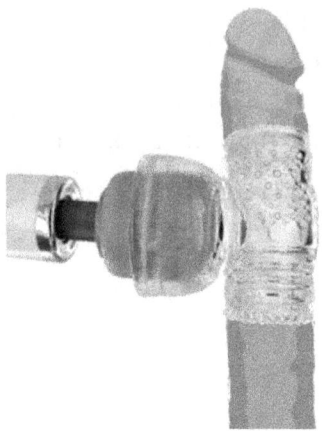

Wand vibrator with attachment and dildo.

Pro Tip 2: A fun setup is having a suction dildo in front of your machine, attached to the floor. You can use a clamp to attach a penis stroker to tip of the machine and turn your sex machine into mechanical stroker. Have it go slow so it feels like you are getting sucked while bouncing on your dildo. When you get close to the climax, remove the stroker and use only the dildo to finish cumming from anal; or remove the stroker and put a dildo on the sex machine to finish.

Hismith Servok and App

There are several other good sex machines available. As of this writing, my favorite is the Hismith Servok machine and its powerful 150W servo motor. Don't get me wrong . . . I still love the old Hismith Premium because it is a reliable work-horse. But the Premium only offers the ability to mechanically adjust the stroke length prior to turning on the machine. It is a manual adjustment, and you can set it anywhere from 0.5" to 6" of thrust depth; however, this is very limiting and tedious.

The newer Hismith Servok is technological dream for prostrainers! This toy takes fuck performance to a whole new level. Unlike traditional crank-link motors that struggle at lower speeds, the motor delivers consistent force under heavy loads across all settings (e.g., fast, slow, shallow, deep strokes). Plus, the real game changer is its ability to adjust both thrust depth and speed directly through an app. This level of precision makes each session highly customizable and fun, allowing you to explore a variety of intensities and rhythms. The only downside is they can be slightly louder compared to the older versions.

The best part about this gadget is its intelligent app-controlled software, seamlessly integrated with your phone. It revolutionizes the entire prostranal experience. The phone app provides comprehensive control over essential thrusting distance, speed, and starting/stopping positions. This means you set everything to your specific preferences. Users can also connect online with partners and the Hismith community to share custom settings and engage in synchronized sessions, making long-distance play an option. For instance, the app allows you to join or create rooms for synchronized experiences. The platform encourages social interaction, enabling users to explore new dimensions of learning and fun together.

The app also offers a selection of pre-set modes designed for various pleasure preferences, making it easy to switch things up when the mood strikes. For those who want to take it a step further, creating personalized routines and curating mode collections is easy. This level of customization not only enriches the user experience, but also allows for adaptive, real-time adjustments. Keep in mind, the app is tricky to navigate at first and needs a bit more development for users. Case in point, it is challenging to create your own predesigned session modes from scratch. That said, the app is incredible because there are user-created modes that are already designed by a community of dedicated users.

Some of the mode sessions go for two minutes, and some for one hour. Some are slow, imitating sensual anal. Others are hard-pounding fuck marathons. There are sessions that escalate gradually, then faster. Some are slow and erratic, so you are always guessing what is coming next.

But beware: there are aggressive modes that rapidly escalate and are bit dangerous because they could tear your hole. Be careful and test them out on the app before you insert! Remember, the app will take a while to figure out, so spend the time to get accustomed before you play.

My favorite part about these new sex machines is that you can create your own patterns and modes or sync your machine so it patterns strokes with music and online porn videos. For example, listening to fast, heavy bass will make it stoke fast and deep versus listening to slower ambient tracks. So many options and moods to play with! Imagine when AI gets integrated into this thing. It's going to get so advanced, it might start giving you relationship advice.

Honorable mention: The **Lovense Sex Machine** is also a solid competitor to the Hismith. I had the chance to see it in action at a trade show, and it definitely impressed. Like others in its class, it features a versatile and robust app for added control and customization. Also known for great customer support.

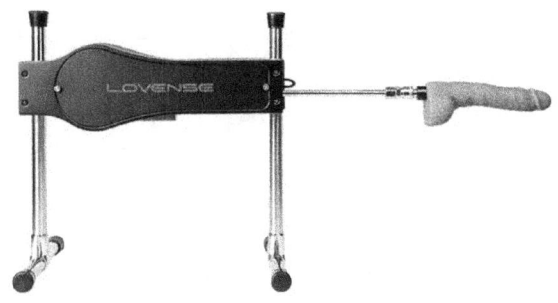

CHAPTER 27

TREMOR, SYBIAN, MOTORBUNNY, LOVEBOTZ . . .

Overview

Have you ever dreamed of being a bull rider? Well, saddle up, partner, because now you can experience the thrill of the ride without leaving your bedroom! Introducing the world of "pleasure saddles" that take your prostate to a whole new level of yee-haw. Designed for ultimate satisfaction, this isn't just a toy; it's your ticket to eight seconds of glory (or maybe 30 minutes, who's counting?). Whether you're a seasoned cowboy or a city slicker, this mechanical marvel will have you shouting "Giddy up!" in no time. Trade the dusty rodeo for your cozy bedroom and let this electronic bull turn your prostate fantasies into reality. Satisfaction guaranteed—or at least a lot of laughs trying! Ride responsibly.

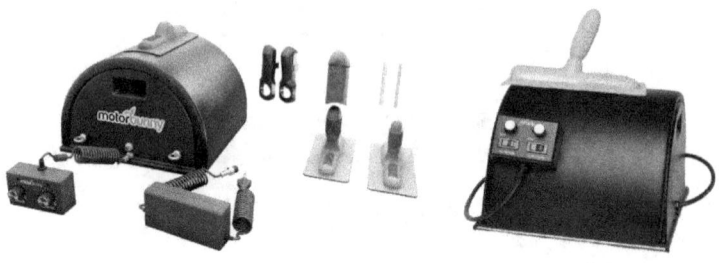

Most of these electric saddles could be classed as A-frame sex machines. You are upright and riding this toy. It adds a whole new element to anal adventure. And if you decide to giddy up and ride one, get ready to spend some money. They range from anywhere between $400-$3,000+ (USD) with all the extras.

They are primarily designed for the clitoris and vagina, making them a bit awkward for prostate play. Nevertheless, these devices can be a helpful and fun way to induce unique anal orgasms. The best ones have thrusting or rotational functionality. Many come with a removable silicone pad and insertable attachments. Not only are they great for riding, but they allow you to rub your cock on the edge of the base plate.

You can purchase attachments. Bad Dragon has several now. And Motorbunny makes great ones as well. I also recommend you get creative instead of splurging on several attachments. You can easily create your own rigs. For instance, I took a shorter P-Spot toy (7 inch) and used a spade drill bit to widen the hole on the base so it fits over the small base nub. I then drilled with a drill bit higher up inside the dildo (creating a 1/8 inch hole), so the rod fits snugly inside. Next, I looped two elastic rings on each end of the base of the dildo and bracket mounts, so it would stay on during the vibrations and the rolling motions.

Most of these sex saddles are heavy, not easy to hide, and difficult to travel with. Some are noisy and loud. And some can quickly cause soreness. Honorable mention goes to Top Drawer Toys for their Box Rocker toy (around $400 USD). This mini rideable toy is quiet, portable and can even be used as a strap on

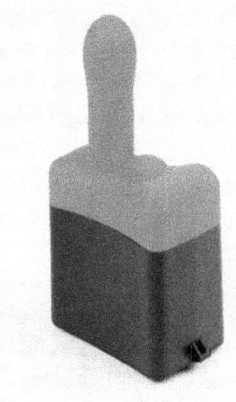

This price, discreteness and power of the Box Rocker makes it a contender in this category.

Pro Tip: Place a sex saddle vertical against a wall or bed so you can put your legs against the wall or on top of the bed (pile-driver position). This beats trying to sit and ride— it keeps the action going without wearing out your legs. Use some pillows to make it more comfortable and enjoy the upside down rodeo!

CHAPTER 28

YOUR CYBORG ASS: TECH AND SEX TOYS

Overview

- Apps are revolutionizing sex tech with remote control play and next-level interactivity.
- Pleasure tracking apps help fine-tune sensations for the ultimate experience.
- Join a new era of connection and customization—build communities, tweak your toys, or even create your own.
- In the prostranal matrix, AI really stands for Anal Intensity.

Welcome to the new sextopia where your smartphone isn't just for scrolling through social media anymore. It's also your gateway to fun sexual experiences! Apps are dialing things up in the sex toy industry, adding a splash of creativity to pleasure. All of these technological breakthroughs mean even more innovative ways to explore and enhance anal play.

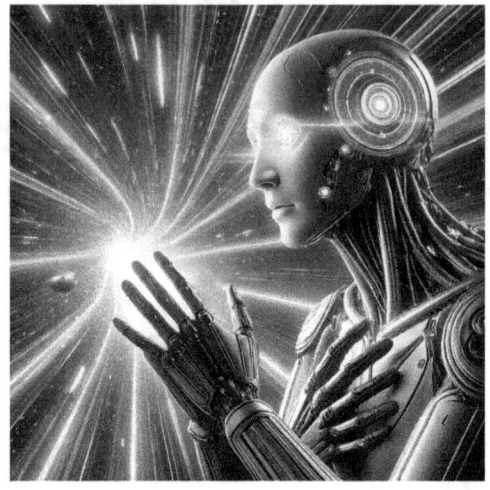

The Remote Control Revolution

Gone are the days of fumbling with buttons while trying to find the right vibe and strokes. Enter app-controlled toys! The We-Vibe Sync O, Lovense Hush 2, AIKYU Remote Vibrator and many more can be controlled from miles away. Picture this: you're out with friends and your partner told you to go out with a butt toy inserted inside you. Your partner is at home and now has the power to wield pleasure right from their phone. With just a tap, they can open the app, then press a button to activate the toy's vibrate or shake function, sending you into waves of ecstasy while you sip your drink. Or you can be on a work trip and video chat with your partner to have some sexy fun, with each of you controlling the action. Talk about a modern twist on long distance relationships! The possibilities are endless.

The Chess Butt Remote Rumor: During a high-profile chess match, there were accusations, internet speculation, and jokes running wild that a famous chess player used a **vibrating device inserted anally** to receive signals from a third party to cheat. This rumor gained traction largely as a meme, highlighting the absurdity of some cheating theories in chess. There's no evidence to support this idea, and it's not taken seriously by the chess community. But the prostrainer community still has questions.

Customization Galore

Apps allow users to tailor their experiences like never before. Want to create the perfect playlist for your solo session? There's an app for that. Do you fancy syncing your toy to the rhythm of your favorite beats? You guessed it—there's an app for that too! With personalized settings and patterns, you can mix and match sensations to find your perfect fit, making every encounter uniquely yours. Check out **xtoys. app** for all the possible configurations. They provide a list of all the toys the app supports and works with, along with detailed guides.

Data-Driven Desire

Who knew data could be so sexy? Some apps come with analytics that track your pleasure patterns. These self-pleasure trackers are like having a personal trainer for your sexual wellness! Forget about guessing what works—users can explore what sensations lead to the best experiences and make informed choices that boost satisfaction. You will need a phone and possibly a fitness tracker or compatible device (e.g., a watch, Fitbit) to use in tandem.

I recommend the following as a starting point:

- **Sex Keeper** – available on both iOS and Android.
- **Nice** – integrates with Apple's HealthKit, and the app offers in-app purchases.
- **Ei Nano** – a free masturbation tracking app. Let's you track toy use or porn, etc. Gender neutral and only available for Android.
- **Coral** – Pricey, but thoughtful, and sex education driven. Available on iOS and Android.
- **Sex Tracker (xTracker)** – another calendar type app for sexual documentation and tracking. Only available on Apple devices.
- **FirmTech** – a smart pleasure tracker app and wearable device that enhances erections and prostate play with real-time performance insights. Available on iOS and Android.

(Check each app to see how it handles your data if you're concerned about privacy.)

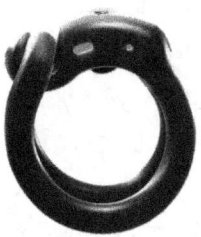

FirmTech's new TechRing might predict your next prostate session before you do.

Pro Tip: The FirmTech TechRing is the next evolution in smart pleasure tracking, combining cutting-edge biometric technology with real-time performance insights. Designed for pleasure optimization, this sleek, wearable device monitors erection quality, duration, and frequency while adapting to individual arousal patterns. TechRing provides users with a data-driven approach to pleasure, allowing them to understand what truly enhances their sexual experience. One of its standout features is its ability to track subtle changes in erection patterns, particularly in response to different forms of stimulation—including prostate play. Whether experimenting with edging, breath control, or prostate massage, users can review real-time feedback on how these techniques affect arousal and stamina. Over time, the TechRing's insights help users fine-tune their pleasure, unlocking deeper levels of sensation. It allows users to experiment with techniques like edging, breath control, and prostate stimulation while tracking the body's responses. This real-time biofeedback makes exploration fun, revealing insights you never knew about your prostate play sessions.

Community and Connection

Many apps are fostering communities where users can share tips, tricks, and experiences. Imagine a virtual support group where everyone's goal is to elevate pleasure and open conversations about desires. It's a safe space to learn and grow, all while connecting with like-minded adventurers. Once you download the sex toy app, see if it has an active community within; or look at finding a Discord server community dedicated to your toy.

Innovative Designs

The marriage of app technology and design has led to some truly bizarre and beautiful creations. From toys that react to your heartbeat to those that sync with virtual reality experiences. The options are as diverse as they are imaginative. It's a playground for grown-ups where creativity knows no bounds!

Apps are changing the way we play. They're redefining the way we feel pleasure and play with each other. If you don't believe me, just scroll through your phone's app store. Don't be surprised if you stumble upon something that makes your mind buzz and insides tingle with intrigue.

If you are highly technology literate, the sky is the limit with your sex toy collection. If you want to go deeper into the possibilities of developing your tech and toys, check out these projects:

- **buttplug.io** – This website gives you open-source standards and software projects for controlling intimate hardware, including sex toys, fucking machines, and more.
- **xtoys.app (guide.xtoys.app)** – If you find the original apps for your toys are limited or difficult to use, this cross-platform app for controlling and automating your toys is your go-to. XToys supports over 700 toys from all major vendors. You can use a variety of control methods to interact with your toys, like on-screen controls, gamepads, VR controllers, voice commands, etc.
- **iostindex.com** – One day this list of toys will disappear. But if you get to see this table of toys, it is quite impressive. Over 800+ toys are shown, but many have been discontinued. It is still fun to peruse and get ideas of what's out there, and what can tie into the Xtoy and Buttplug maker space.

Who knows, maybe one day there will be a GitHub copycat called ButtHub—a platform that provides tools for version control and collaboration, allowing developers to host, review, and manage code repositories for anal driven tech projects. One can dream . . .

CHAPTER 29

GOING ANALOG: SEAT ROCKERS, GLIDERS, BOUNCERS, CUSHIONS, SWINGS, BALLS BIKES . . .

Overview

- Bouncers, cushions, and swings are ready-to-buy gear but need a little physical effort and creativity to maximize their potential.
- Explore DIY toys and contraptions ideas to customize your prostate play experience.
- Please refrain from stealing your grandmother's walker to build an anal pleasuring device.

Can you imagine what they probably came up with in the 19th century before reliable electricity and batteries? Picture a steampunk-inspired contraption, complete with levers, gears, and maybe even a hand crank. Some poor soul probably had to pedal a wooden bike in their parlor to get the thing going, while trying to maintain a straight face as they called it "therapeutic exercise". Let's be honest, those Victorian inventors might have been onto something, but thank goodness we've swapped clunky gadgets and coal-powered machinery for smoother, more modern analog options!

In a world where everything seems to have a battery, motor, or app, sometimes it's refreshing to go back to basics. Enter manual-powered prostate toys—the ultimate "analog" experience for those who want to combine pleasure with a little physical effort. These contraptions rely on your body's own strength, movement, and gravity to create stimulation. Forget simply pushing a button or plugging in a cord; with these tools, *you* are the motor!

This section dives into the world of manual devices that even Stewie Griffin, Rick Sanchez, and MacGyver would be proud of.

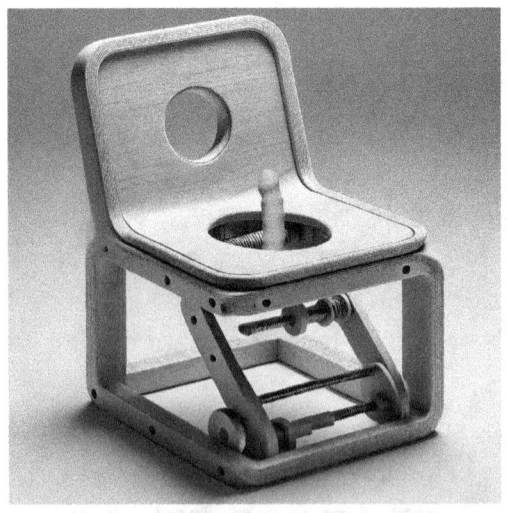

The image shown here could be the future office chair of Prostranal Headquarters.

Seat rockers and gliders

In *Burn After Reading*, George Clooney's character, Harry, shows off a homemade sex chair to Frances McDormand, rocking it with a grin. It's funny, but it points to a truth: seat rockers and gliders are kinky furniture for some people. These aren't just movie props—they blend clever design with playful vibes.

Self-powered sex machines that are controlled by rocking your body back and forth or bouncing up and down on a sex toy (e.g., dildo). With every movement, there's a thrust and filling sensation that your toy brings. A seat rocker or glider is a specialized piece of sex furniture. You operate the speed and depth of penetration by using your legs, or the device, for leverage. All of these manual devices provide different forms of hands-free stimulation. Your movements can convert powerful thrusts into convulsive anal orgasms. This is for those into deep penetrative fun! Because you're in control of the thrust and penetration, it makes for the ultimate sex partner. Most manual rocker/glider sex setups can be used with dildos, probes, and vibrators. This gives you a wide variety of options.

Adjustable settings offer customizable depth and penetration for enhanced stimulation. Control is somewhat simple—the more you grind your hips, the better the prostate thrusts. Best of all, these are much quieter than their electronic alternatives. But keep in mind, that these devices typically require physical exertion. Depending on your setup, you will probably get a workout and tire fast. Some swear they are the best anal-only orgasms achieved; but for most, it is not guaranteed and can be tricky. The cost of these sex seats/gliders is high, anywhere from $500 - $3,000+ (USD). If you explore on **FetLife**, you might be able to find one or have one custom built. **Amazon, eBay** and **Etsy** are also good places to look. There are even plans available for you to build your own at **funkyrocker.com.**

Bouncing benches

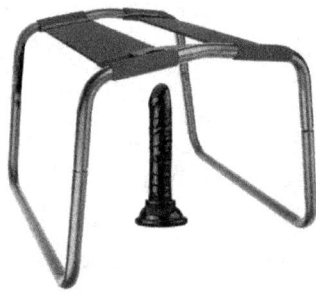

If you are looking for a workout and a sex toy, this will make you break a sweat. They usually come with steel frames and have elastic seating, perfect for bouncing. They are lightweight but strong, and can easily be taken apart and stored out of sight, unlike a sex chair.

You just lift your hips up and down and bounce away on your favorite dildo. You will need to adjust the angle of the dildo so you can enjoy different positions and find your sweet spot angled forward, leaned back, facing front, or reversing your position. As with most of these "bouncing furniture novelties", you will need to be in good shape because of the physical exercise involved to reach an anal orgasm.

Some people love to be covered in sweat and get a good workout that mimics sex. Others prefer to let electricity do all the work. I have bad knees, so this one went straight to the Goodwill donation after I purchased it. I wonder if they were ever able to figure out what it was.

Sex cushions/sex saddle toy mounts

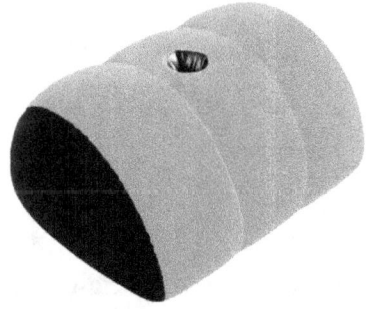

Entertaining if you are on a budget. Most sex cushions are made from high-density foam that supports your body during grinding and pumping playtime. Many have removable covers that are water-resistant to make cleanup and maintenance easy. There are also inflatable pillows that are ideal for travel. Get one that has a toy slot to hold your favorite dildo or vibrator for hands-free fun. Sex pillows let you explore new angles and options with anal play, all while getting more comfortable and finding deeper penetration. They are also great to use with partners. Like bouncing benches, they are easy to stow away when not in use.

Sex swings

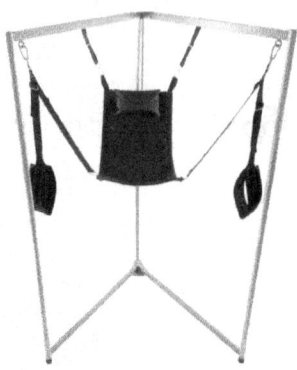

Out of all the options mentioned in this section, you cannot go wrong with a good sex swing, especially since you can use it with a partner outside of solo-prostate play. They're fun for those who want to try suspended positions and find the best angle with the least amount of effort. They are best to use with a sex machine. But you can use it with just a toy (dildo or vibrator) and rock back and forth manually.

Many swings come with restraints and attachments to dial-in your play. But be very careful if you are using a swing that mounts into the ceiling! Read the manual thoroughly and follow the manufacturer's instructions carefully. There are also door swing varieties that are not permanent, are travel-friendly, and far easier to mount. Or buy a yoga swing and use it as a sex sling.

Exercise balls

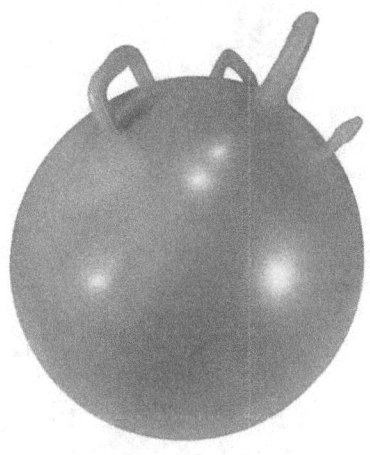

The exercise balls with suction dildos are another stop along the anal highway. You can buy one that already has dildos built in; referred to as a "dildo ball". This takes anal workouts to another level—the perfect combination of core and leg exercise mixed with pleasure. A possible downside is they are kind of hard to store and will make for an awkward conversation if your mom went into your closet or garage and found it. Over-inflation is risky since this could damage or pop the ball.

Not every toy is designed to fit. If you buy a dildo ball, the dildos might not be big enough, or too big. Suction dildos on exercise balls fall off easily and are hard to keep mounted. Also, they can be tricky to clean—and you do need to clean them thoroughly after every use to eliminate germs and bacteria. You also might not be the right height or weight to enjoy them.

Bikes, and the Like

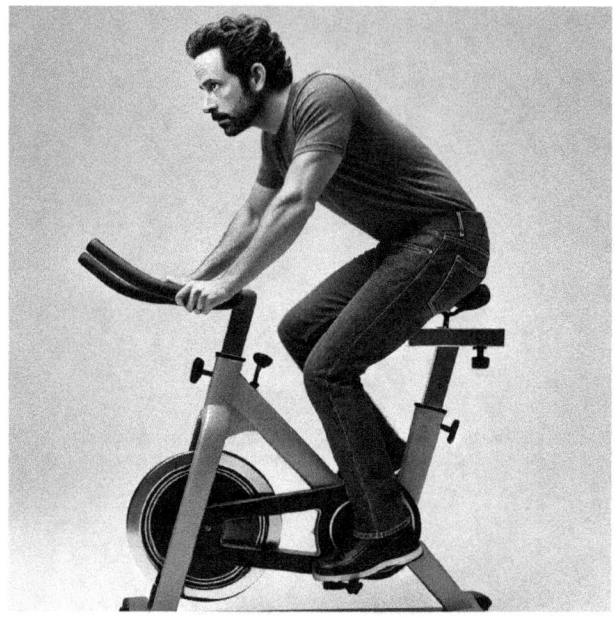

The TV show It's Always Sunny in Philadelphia revealed Mac's "Ass-Pounder 4000". This isn't far-fetched as there are "engineer" pros-trainers who go to thrift stores and modify old exercise equipment.

Look into making your own sex contraptions built from old bikes, elliptical machines, rowing machines, etc. If you are mechanically inclined, there are plenty of websites that showcase DIY builds, providing directions and diagrams. There are several options to creating the perfect device, and much of it can be built using items you may already own.

CHAPTER 30

THE PERFECT COMBINATION: BRINGING IT ALL TOGETHER

Overview

- Review all the chapters with a complete break-down of key concepts.
- Apply what you've learned—experiment, refine, and elevate your experience.
- At this point, your ass, mind, or eyes are probably exhausted from this renegade adventure. Or maybe you're just stressing about where to hide this book from your roommate or family. First-world problems, am I right?

In my experience, there is no perfect path with prostate play. Instead, think of this book like a recipe collection: Each chapter is a delicious dish on its own, but when you combine them, you create the ultimate feast. Now, it's time to bring all those flavors together and create your own menu.

The **Staircase** chapter explained the foundation of learning and progressing, step by step. Harness the creative power of your mind to combine every arousal amplification technique you learned into something new and personal. Every day you should be inching forward with your goals; doing your best to rewire, strengthen and transform your body into a finely tuned pleasure machine. You are creating an alignment between intention and action, in order to create the perfect conditions for success.

You now have all tools—your A-less, Mindgasm and PAT! Combine this with your newfound love for breathwork, sound arousal, hypnosis, etc., and you are wielding a force that transcends the physical. Without touch, you can now activate arousal on your perineum, prostate, penis, nipples, scrotum, and anus. You now can build your skills to mix and match these techniques, creating the perfect framework for pleasure. The best part? There's no limit to how much you can refine, explore, and enjoy this process. Dream the endless!

Your newfound knowledge will also help you find equipment that gets you to the top of your mountain. By creatively combining prostate techniques and configuring sex toys, you can unlock a world of exciting possibilities. It can be as simple as you want it to be. Or complex as a Rube Goldberg machine. This customization allows you to prioritize your unique preferences, making playtime more exciting and functional. Safely using sex equipment with creativity, will take your orgasms even higher!

And at the heart of all this exploration is prostate health and safety, because without a solid foundation, the house doesn't stand. You've learned the importance of regular checkups, of listening to your body and your doctor. And of taking care of your health—not just for the here and now, but for the long haul. After all, what's the point of unlocking the secrets of pleasure if you're not around to enjoy them, or suffering in a hospital?

So here you are, standing at the edge of the last chapters—not just in this book, but in your old life. A new you is emerging. Belief, acceptance, and surrender are the graffiti scrawled across the shell of your former self. It's now a part of your DNA. Take a moment to clearly define your intention and reaffirm your declaration again. Believe that you can experience prostate orgasms. Flood yourself with positive thinking daily. Be a fierce soldier in the battle to defeat the old self. Maintain this progress to build your flow.

As a dedicated prostrainer, it's time to dive even deeper into your journey of self-discovery. Become your own interviewer and ask yourself hard questions everyday: How can I get more creative? What else do I need to learn? How can I truly meet my body's needs? Embrace curiosity and be open to exploring new techniques. Think outside the box as you continue to evolve your prostate practice. Growth happens when you step out of your comfort zone, shake up your routine and challenge your limits. Don't be afraid to push the boundaries of what you thought was possible.

The perfect combination isn't about perfection; it's about blending wonder, adaptation, and a healthy dose of humor into your journey. Don't be afraid to laugh at yourself. Be bold, be playful, and most importantly, be kind to your future prostate. You've created a roadmap to pleasure that's uniquely your own. Now go out there and live it. You've earned it. There is no shame—only pleasure going forward!

CHAPTER 31

PROSTATE TALES FROM THE KINK

Overview

Every kink has its own rhythm, and what gets one person turned on might leave another feeling grossed out. As humans, we especially learn through storytelling, finding pieces of ourselves in others' journeys. Hence, I've gathered stories that run the spectrum—from deeply philosophical viewpoints to downright juicy and hot tales. Be ready for everything. Dive in, and maybe you'll find one that resonates with your own beat . . . or inspires you. And who knows? By the end, you might just have a story or two of your own to tell for the next book.

Collected and curated anal confessions to inspire and arouse you . . .

Never Settling

"I have been practicing prostate massage for many years and had my first Super-O a long time ago. Even to this day, it still feels like I am learning something new. Sometimes the orgasms are incredibly mental, spiritual, or physical. It depends on my mood. And somehow, they still feel as powerful as the first ones. I will never forget the first Super-O. It terrified me because it felt so great and rocked my world!

Am I different from before I started? I still have penile orgasms, but less than before I learned to cum from my prostate. Now, I edge more and ejaculate less. I changed in other ways, too. It altered my self-awareness and sexuality. I'm more in touch with my physical and emotional self now. It hasn't radically changed my outlook on the world; instead, I have transcended into more of a spiritual being. It has also opened me up to being more understanding of others and their kinks and personal lifestyles. I had a very closed mind before all of this prostate stuff and mostly saw the world in "black and white".

Best of all, my sex life improved with my partner. We have more fun in bed, and longer, more meaningful sex that can go on all night. I even believe it made me fantasize less about sleeping with other partners. I feel more fulfilled now and wouldn't want to waste my time and pleasure with someone else. It's really hard to find a woman who is open about exploring the "dark arts" of prostate play.

My early years of seeking anal orgasms, however, were not easy ones. It was challenging to just stop masturbating with my hand and try to figure out how to play with my ass. It was always a gratification battle for me. After some time, I learned that I could either substantially alter my life with super-orgasmic pleasure or settle for lower-quality penile orgasms. It went slowly facing these choices, and I finally figured out a way to have as much of both as possible. There's often a better path waiting—you just probably haven't discovered it yet. So keep looking for it rather than settling for the choice that is ordinary and comfortable. Prostate play is the next level. It's not exactly time travel or a near-death experience, but it comes pretty close."

—Xander

Edging to Assgasm

"My first assgasm happened when I was edging. I achieved it by stimulating my frenulum at the same time as I was rocking back and forth on an anal plug that hit my P-Spot. It was a padded stool, and I was almost standing, which is my favorite position. I sat on the large butt plug, rocking back and forth for 15 minutes. As soon as the anal pleasure came, I teased and tickled my head close to cumming several times. Then I stopped touching myself and finally pushed myself over the edge with only the butt plug. I started to learn the separation between penile and anal orgasms, and how to bridge them. I experimented with edging for some time to get a deeper understanding of how my body worked. By doing this daily, it became easier to finally cum from just anal with no edging.

I learned that when I start feeling a contraction, I don't go deeper, harder, or faster. I just keep doing the thing that brought me these contractions. Over and over again, I keep the same movement, speed, and angle. With a dildo, I love long and slow hard strokes with a lot of pressure on my prostate; flicking it feels like it is hooking along my anal cavity. I get these incredibly intense contractions that force my prostate to rub harder against the thrusting toy. Reality lags like a glitch in the matrix. I start to leave my body. It's like I am dreaming. Somehow, I keep at it, repeating the motion, and fucking myself, feeling the waves and contractions. It's the ultimate pleasure. Every time I cum, I still think, *Is this really what women feel like when they hit their G-Spot and have convulsive orgasms?* I look down at my penis and see cum. I'm squirting like a girl. My ass feels like a pussy, and my cock's head feels like a clit.

Now the hardest part is to not want an assgasm every day. It's like I woke up one day and had an entirely new genitalia installed. I feel like I am going through puberty again."

—Thomas

To Pee or Not to Pee

"I was really horny one day, so I got out my prostate wand. I lubed it up, inserted the smaller stainless-steel end into me, and started to wake up my prostate. It was instant pleasure indeed, with the right angle sending tremors through my body. I sped up and was hitting my prostate so fast that I felt a sudden but pleasurable feeling like needing to pee. I experienced this before when playing with my prostate, but not like this intensity. It was an uncontrollable need to pee, but with deep anal pleasure the more I resisted peeing. I was scared and stopped. But it didn't prevent my body from shaking and trembling.

I then started rubbing my prostate again until I got to the same predicament. I stopped and did it again and again, over and over. At one point, I was moving the wand in and out, fucking myself so hard and fast that I finally squirted clear and milky fluids from the tip of my penis. The sensations were like nothing I'd experienced before, and they were causing me to cry out and shake. I lay there in a puddle, confused and drained.

But I was still very horny. So I used the larger end of my wand and started again. My ass felt so swollen that I didn't think it would fit in my hole this time. It was intimidating—I never had anything inside me this big. But I got it in and proceeded to fuck my ass hard and fast again. The sensations were even stronger this time! The waves of pleasure were coursing through me, and I finally gave in to them. This time instead of pee and prostatic fluid, I was cumming everywhere! I was so turned on and curious that I tasted my cum for the first time. It was so sweet and actually tasted good that I ate it all up in a crazed state of lust. I'd never felt like such an animal before.

That day, I learned that if I can get over the challenge of needing to pee, I could cum. That was my first experience cumming from anal. It took me a while to surrender, but once I let go of control, I was finally able to orgasm. It's such an amazing and intense feeling. I wish everyone I know could experience it. I'm just too scared to tell my guy friends that everyone deserves to get the cum fucked out of them by having their prostate rubbed."

—Jordy

Awaking the Anal Dragon

"After a year of using a sex machine, I decided to carve an Aneros-like toy out of wood. When I finished, it looked pretty underwhelming. But I was determined to make it work. I quickly learned there are countless ways to experience pleasure, whether it's through touching your erogenous zones, massaging larger muscle groups, teasing your nipples, or exploring the sensitive area between the testes and the tailbone. The first couple days, I had lots of exciting feelings, erections, and even some leaking. I wore a monitor to see what my heart rate would be along the way and see how high I could get it. My heart rate typically peaks at 132 beats per minute (bpm) when I orgasm. With the wooden prostate massager and all the self-touching, I was doing, it got me close to 122 bpm. Not bad!

Into this journey, I kept a log and journal to track everything. I started to figure out the secrets of my internal spots by focusing on the sensations that the external stimulation awakened throughout my body. I could feel deep pleasure with my kegels. I started lightly contracting and pushing the toy along my prostate. The buildup was incredible. There were some mild waves and spasms. I had a few mild dry orgasms for the first time. My belly and legs clenched hard during these peaks. After a while of shaking, I was out of breath and feeling almost a post-orgasm sensation even though I did not ejaculate. This was a good start!

I relaxed a minute and tried to repeat. Again, I was

gently rubbing my body wherever it felt sensitive. My hands followed the pleasure. Soon, I got more excited and focused on lightly rubbing my nipples while using my other hand to manually stimulate my prostate with the toy—wiggling it in and out, rotating it, and experimenting with different motions. A thundering orgasm washed over me with even more shaking, clenching, and heavy breathing. It lasted much longer than any so far during this session. I rode that wave of pleasure all the way to the shore.

I rinsed and repeated this routine for hours. My heart rate monitor registered readings near 154 bpm during one Super-O. The pleasure was so intense I lost track of time and barely noticed the pool of fluids on my stomach. Despite not achieving an official hands-free wet orgasm, it didn't bother me. Draining my prostate was an incredible experience, leaving me with an electrifying sensation afterward. My body tingled with energy, a feeling that lasted into the next day.

Over time, I've continued this process once or twice a week, with good outcomes. Most of these sessions lead to my first dry orgasm within 4 minutes. I then prolong the pleasure as much as possible. The shortest session lasted around 30 minutes, featuring multiple orgasms, some with just brief recovery intervals, and a few feeling unending even after several breathless minutes.

Today marked my longest session, slightly surpassing 4 hours, prompting me to document the experience in my journal. This session happened in two phases. The first was an extended version of my previous attempts. It was full of intense shaking, clenching, and lots of fluid release. Roughly an hour later, my body felt tired and somewhat sore. As I stretched my legs to find relief and savor the post-orgasmic calm, an accidental movement triggered another prostate orgasm, setting off another surge of intense involuntary contractions. Once again, I was caught in back-to-back, minute-long orgasms, completely powerless to stop them. Each time I assumed it was ending, even the slightest motion brought on another wave of overwhelming full-body shakes. It was 8.5 on the anal Richter scale. I happily surrendered, utterly wrecked by pleasure, amazed at how calm my breathing stayed and how completely relaxed my body felt throughout it all. This was a completely new experience for me.

Even after an additional 42 minutes of uninterrupted pleasure, my mind had barely focused on my cock. I almost forgot it was even there! That's when I decided to rub the head and wake it up. In seconds, I felt the familiar sensation of a wet orgasm building, even though it remained soft the entire time. I continued rubbing, jerking, and pinching until I finally started to ejaculate. But it wasn't a standard release. It was an unexpected surge of fluids—a full-on "peegasm." I soaked myself and continued stroking until another wave of tremors swept over me, turning into a real penis ejaculation. I laid in my own wet mess, gasping for breath, tingling with sensations, and rubbing the fluids all over myself like some deranged abstract painter.

I missed an important appointment that afternoon, but I didn't mind. It was the most pleasurable memory of my prostate journey, and worth every minute of it."

—Rehdi

I Came My First Time

"I first discovered anal bliss with a large dildo that I bought at a sex shop when I was younger. I always enjoyed the feeling of ass play with my finger, or homemade objects, inside me when I masturbated. But the dildo going in and out of me while stroking my cock made my whole body feel like it was levitating. The instant it went inside me, I felt something change. I never experienced this before and loved it. These new sensations felt like my cock was going to cum. I played with the dildo for a few minutes and grabbed my cock at the same time, stoking slowly because it seemed like I was going cum so fast. Within seconds, I stopped playing with myself and used both hands to hammer the dildo into me as fast as possible. I quickly felt involutaries, reached a gentle anal orgasm and felt my ass pulsating. I kept the dildo inside and started fucking myself all over again. This led to having several more climaxes until the final one washed the cum out of me like nothing I've ever felt before. Anal orgasms sometimes feel like you're cumming out of your eyeballs, heart and toes.

There was no going back to regular masturbation after this experience. After an anal orgasm, normal (hand) penile orgasms became meaningless to me. Nothing even comes close to the pleasure that an anal orgasm gives me."

—Garret

No Limit

"I don't want to sound like a certain Jedi Master, but . . .

anticipate being deceived early along the way of your path. You might believe that you have never cum as hard once you start with your first prostate orgasms—only to reach higher levels of pleasure weeks and months later. Whether it is a P-Gasm or Super-O, there is no ceiling to prostate pleasure. The "best case" can be exceeded on the upside.

And there are many ways to level up as you climb this staircase. I've been raising the vibe through exploring the power of my mind: Visualization of cumming, mental imagination of stimulation, and contracting my pelvic floor muscles. Sometimes I start with my toys and touch my cock to get started. But I force myself to stop, then use the force of my mind and will power with intention to keep the pleasure going. This didn't mean I stopped having sessions with my other toys and rigs. One day I decided to see how I could incorporate my mind, rather than it being only physical. This is when the magic started for me!

You have to adjust your practices when you are on this long journey to unlock your prostate. It's not until you get to those basic, orgasmic lessons in prostate play that it gets more subtle and fine. Then there'll be moments of clarity to navigate into this unknown territory. One day, a door just opens, and what once felt like holding a candle in your hand transforms into the warmth of a winter sunset on your face—slow, lingering, and endlessly golden.

It is about being able to let go of your control and sur-rendering. Not only to your muscles and breath, but total disintegration of the mind. Once you do this, you'll have that first breakthrough session of never-ending pleasure. Time will deceive you! It could last 15 minutes to an hour, but you won't know it. Even if there was a clock in your room, it wouldn't matter. Each orgasm crashes over the other. It feels like there is no beginning or end. It is the ultimate quantum rush. You are in it: The flow of *shakti*, life, energy. You just become lost in circular breath, writhing in rapture, moaning, maybe screaming, and definitely shaking like an epileptic hugging someone with Parkinson's disease.

This type of Super-O experience is so powerful that you'll never be the same. It'll be in your mind for days. Some see it as powerful as an *Ayahuasca* ceremony, or similar to a near death experience. As you learn to repeat this over and over, your inner confidence grows, and you see that ceiling of pleasure disappear. This magic will cross over into your normal life as well. You'll be changed and there is no going back.

If you feel like you have plateaued in your practice, do not despair. Maybe take a break for a few days or weeks. But rest assured, the best is yet to come, and you are closer than you think."

—Wayne

The Mental Journey

"Exploring my own depths has been a slow and indulgent voyage. Before Mindgasm, my focus was only on instant gratification—just the usual manual masturbation and a little prostate exploration. I had this notion that I might stumble upon the right partner who'd be up for entering anal play territory with me. It's evident that everything before Mindgasm was a rather self-centered narrative. Eventually, the meaningful lessons flowed from my Mindgasm experience. A symphony of discoveries echoed through, including the art of tuning into my body's needs and possibilities, distinguishing between moods that sync and those that diverge. Pleasure escalated beyond the realms of mere physicality, engaging the mind and prostate as one.

It transformed me into a more complete and harmonious sexual being, finely attuned to the cadence of my own body, and those who share my orbit. The allure here is its ceaseless evolution and fluidity, a continuum of learning that unveils limitless perspectives, inventive techniques, and sensations that expand the senses. This entire escapade is an odyssey, extending as far as my desires dare to chart.

For me, Mindgasm gave me unlimited sensations, an elixir of invincibility coursing through my veins. At first, I believed that I had reached the peak of sexual knowledge. Oh, how childlike I was! Time and exchanges with others in the prostate community deflated that egocentric balloon. I must have been quite the pest, asking about every possible detail about anal orgasms to everyone. Lucky for me, they endured and answered my endless questions. And once I had my first mind orgasm, the path to enlightenment truly started."

—Nathaniel

Finding the Manhole

"I was driving one day and saw several construction signs at the intersection of the road: "Do not Enter", "Left Turn Only", "Detour", etc. Hidden behind them was a manhole that was barely visible.

It dawned on me that this was what it was like for me to learn to cum from anal. I had to remove all the road signs, figure out where the entrance was, how to open the manhole cover and climb down the stairs. Inside this space, I found that there was a speakeasy of pleasure. There were intricate mechanical gears, there was a sanctuary . . .

I had to learn how to become an explorer and engineer, how to become intoxicated (aka "an analholic") and how to spiritually awaken. And once I did, there was no turning back. Nothing again can ever stop me from finding this pleasure palace or keep me away from it."

—Franky

A Detonation of Sexual Energy

"My prostate workshop retreats have always brought great conversations. One that stands out is with a co-facilitator and good friend. Brad had been contemplating our conversations with the group the day before. We spent two days during this retreat in Mexico trying to take everyone's backgrounds and experience into account.

One participant became passionate defending his method that allowed him to easily cum from anal. He boasted it was the best and only way to climax. Brad had considered responding to this argument about whether one needed to perform penis play during prostate sessions, and whether or not you even needed to directly stimulate the prostate.

This brought up a long discussion on Tantra/Taoist aspects around prostate pleasure and sexual energy. As a co-presenter, he knew his stuff. Brad set out to thoughtfully explore this subject from his own perspective, hoping to inspire others to look beyond their current practices and break through their perceived limitations.

Since embarking on his path three years ago, Brad had studied these topics in great detail, and he read voraciously. He was one of the first participants of my earlier workshops. He quickly transformed his perception of sexual pleasure, resulting in personal life changes: career, marriage, and relationships with others. He admitted to the group that if someone had told him three years prior about the boundless pleasure and personal breakthroughs that come from prostate play, he would have dismissed them and thought they were "hitting on him" or were crazy. But Brad now knew that humans possess the capability to experience incredibly intense levels of pleasure that can transcend into the spiritual realm.

Brad became a Joe Dispenza disciple as well during his transformation. He strongly believed in the untapped potential of the human brain. He explained in his lecture that there are unmapped and untapped areas across the brain, typically restricted due to trauma, lack of knowledge, societal norms, and so on.

With this, Brad proposed to the group accessing these "off-limits" brain areas, and venture beyond the boundaries of ones' own brain and spirit. He likened it to us needing to be an oil or gold explorer. We needed to set out and seek the resources of "potential pleasure". More importantly, to not stop no matter what you find.

Once he had shared this foundation to the group, Brad moved on to explain how to redefine pleasure, exploring mindfulness through basic meditation techniques, and incorporating various breathing exercises, to relax and build this untapped sexual energy. By amalgamating mindfulness, relaxation, deep breathing, and techniques to move sexual energy, Brad experienced a rejuvenation of his body. He welcomed a plethora of new sensations that fueled heightened sexual energy and pleasure. He shared his testament, and moved the group to full attention, generating several questions.

Brad suggested diverging from traditional pleasure pathways, redirecting focus toward newly discovered methods. He emphasized that while stimulation to the penis wasn't mandatory, it could serve as an additional channel, if needed. But it should not be a means to an end or final destination. Brad urged a retraining of the brain away from conventional pleasure pathways leading to traditional ejaculatory orgasms. He advocated for embracing diverse forms of pleasure, encouraging sensuality through gentle touches and massages across the body, chanting, long meditations, and Tantra/Chi exercises. His key message revolved around relaxation, being present in the moment, and embracing any and all forms of pleasure that one encounters, while not ignoring the subtle streams of pleasure often overlooked. Being attuned to even the smallest sensations could expand one's pleasure pathways and open a new spiritual gateway.

Brad acknowledged that this journey demanded time, practice, and experimentation. He stressed the importance of allowing oneself to deeply relax for this divine sexual experience to arrive. He believed that such exploration would ultimately create a positive circle of energy, endlessly intensifying arousal. This loop would trigger a nuclear fission of pleasure—an eruption of sensation unlike anything felt before.

Brad knew that learning these ancient techniques would change the way we view and experience pleasure. It also changes your life forever. The workshops we conducted weren't just events; they were our gift to the public, a heartfelt dedication, and our purpose-driven calling. Through sexuality, we aimed to cultivate transformative, uplifting, and restorative encounters, no matter how difficult the conversation."

—Elo

Anal Hook Up: Uno Reverse

"A long time ago, I met a woman at a bar close to my apartment. She was actually wearing a T-shirt that said, "I Love Anal". We hit it off right away, and after chatting and playing pool, I asked her, "Do you also like spanking?"

She bent over, slapped her butt and said, "Of course I do!"

There haven't been many times in my life where this type of scenario happened, so I knew it was going to be a fun time.

When she showed up at my door the next evening, she professed her deep love for hard spankings and anal sex. It wasn't long before we were in the bedroom exploring these topics in real time. We became FWBs and our sex encounters got better and better over time.

One night she surprised me by asking, "Have you ever been fucked in the ass?"

I replied, "I've had fingers and a toy up my ass once,

but never have I been fucked by a woman."

She opened her handbag and pulled out a strap-on kit, explaining, "Well, I'm going to bend you over tonight, spank you, and then fuck you in the ass. Okay?"

I was so excited to hear these words from a woman for the first time in my life that I could feel the precum form. But honestly, I didn't think I'd really enjoy it. I figured that after a few minutes I'd end up laughing and ruining the role-play.

After some preparation and spanking, she turned me around and put me on my hands and knees. I glanced back a few times, watching her adjust the harness and lube up the head of the massive cock.

Like a nurse, she told me, "You're going to feel a slight prick," as she shuffled in closer behind me with her anal needle. I gladly spread my cheeks, and she put the head inside my tight hole. Immediately, I tensed up and the pain grew. It felt hot and like someone ripped off a bandage inside my asshole.

I whimpered and she asked me if I was alright, recommending, "You just need to relax more, and then it'll start to feel good."

She helped by reaching around to stroke me while massaging my back with her other hand. As she teased, I began to enjoy the slow thrusts of the dildo. She pushed deeper the more I moaned. After a few moments, I arched my back and started to take over, riding it in bliss. Her long, thick cock filled me with joy. It felt like my hole was sucking her cock like a hungry, slutty mouth.

There was a moment when I panicked because it felt like I was going to shit myself. She laughed and started spanking my ass, talking obscenely to me. After a while, she picked up her pace, fucking me harder and faster. She squirted more lube above my ass crack and let it drip onto her toy. I loved it and wanted more. My ass responded by aggressively shoving back into her thrusts. It was fascinating to be on the other side of the sword.

Instantly, as if she knew it would happen, she found my P-Spot and honed in with even deeper and harder thrusts. It only lasted a minute until I shot cum all over the bed. She didn't even care! She just pulled it out for a few seconds to use the cum as lube and then stuck it back in, making me cum again a few minutes later.

I looked down and could see my cock swinging wildly shooting cum everywhere. It was my first anal orgasm, and it shattered me. Finally, I collapsed on the bed and was unable to move.

She spooned me, lightly caressed my face and body, and cooed, "You were such a good whore tonight. I bet you're going to want to be fucked like that from now on."

It was a totally mind-blowing experience. Not only was my ass shattered, but my sense of gender and role was transformed forever."

—Jaime

CHAPTER 32

TALE END

Overview

More prostrainer confessions—the kinkier, the better. Things are about to get much spicier!

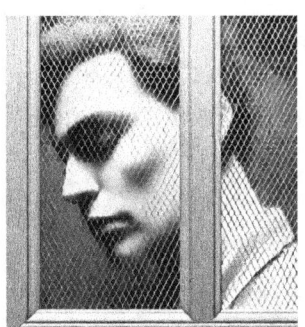

Try It . . . You'll Like It

"It felt like a school science project at times. Like I was back in 8th grade trying to make a volcano diorama. But instead of baking soda and vinegar, I was chasing the prostate dragon with a dildo and lube. It wasn't easy, but eventually, I figured it out.

I never quit—no matter how tough it got, I kept push-ing. I messed around with all kinds of tools: hard, soft, big, small, straight, curved, you name it. I switched up how I used them—straight on, angled, front, back, whatever felt right. I tried every position in the book: flat on my back, on all fours, squatting, standing. I played with speeds, fast and slow, and powered through even when it seemed pointless. Bottom line? I didn't stop.

What worked best for me might not be the same for you. I found that I preferred a thicker, and more flexible dildo. The most important thing for me was the angle. Going straight in didn't do much. It's hard to explain, but when I'm in the shower and the dildo is on the wall, placed a bit high so it goes down when it enters me, the dildo presses on my prostate with each movement. For me, the best feeling comes when the head almost slips out each time, and not too deep, and the "taint" (perineum) feels like it is getting squeezed.

Stimulating the prostate is a subtle feeling at first. You have to pay close attention to the things you don't notice. Never touch your penis, as it could be too distracting. Avoid methods that require too much effort, like holding your toys—instead, use an electronic device designed to stay in place. Sex machines rule!

You want to build up fluid in the prostate to increase feelings of pleasure. When you rub or hit the prostate, it's better to start slow. Get that area primed. After a while, you will have orgasms and you will release prostate fluid.

If you don't feel anything, practice more. You can never have enough playtime if you are not sore! Poke around gently when you're relaxed and horny. Those two extremes teach you a lot about your prostate. The feeling you are looking for is like a tingling in your tummy. If it's like an itch. A good itch. Keep scratching it.

If you do hit your P-Spot right, you'll feel the pleasure waves spread throughout your body. Practice can make this feeling stronger, and lead to a dry prostate orgasm. Dry ones lead to wet ones. And wet ones lead to heaven.

If you're stuck, try new things. Change positions, speeds, toys, and maybe zip codes. Explore different sensations to figure out what feels good and always take your time to orgasm. Cancel any appointments with the Governor for that day.

Anal, anal, and more anal is the way to get used to anal. Just as prostate, prostate, and prostate gets you to more prostate orgasms. Frequency is the best teacher because the more you do it the better you become. Get out there and spread your hole . . . then practice, practice, practice until you are sore! Become an anal whore with your toys!

Don't over-stress it. An anal orgasm needs mental focus too. Put less pressure on yourself and enjoy the moment. Yell "Shit!" and "Fuck!" at the ceiling or house plant when you need to blow some steam. Focus on what you find feels nice rather than what you read is *supposed* to feel good. It is just a process of elimination. Scream "Shit!" and "Fuck!" at the ceiling or house plant when you finally erupt and cum. Say you're sorry to the house plant when you are done."

—Jake

CTRL ALT DELETE

"Once I realized that my need for control was holding me back, I became like a balloon and floated away from the shackles of my mind and body. It was the tiniest things that weighed me down in life I realized. I was scared to let go and fully surrender to experiences. From the smallest clenches when the toy was in me, to the desire to do everything the "right way", I needed to LET ALL OF IT GO.

My training began with teaching myself how to do this while learning to control my breath. That is when I started to feel my prostate come alive. I found the spot. After the tingles set in, the warmth followed. My prostate was happy and laughing for the first time in my life. The pleasure grew into waves, sometimes overlapping, and like a tsunami. My mind went blank. I eventually lost control of my breathing and thoughts. I only remember the sweat dripping down my thighs and the back of my spine. I couldn't stop or control anything. The incredible pleasure lasted for minutes, then returned even stronger. I started to hallucinate, becoming vocal while convulsing. The body just takes over. It's like dying.

After the orgasm, I resurrected from the dead. I loved the deeply gratifying afterglow and how it lingered for so long. I stayed aroused, fully satisfied, and in an incredibly good mood after my first Super-O.

Unlike the fatigue and listlessness I often feel after penile orgasms, anal orgasms leave me energized and uplifted. I feel like Super-Os open up my heart more and more. Life energy gushes everywhere around me. I walk outside feeling superhuman, more confident and alive!"

—Max

I Can Feel It Coming (In the Air Tonight, Oh Lord!)

"It took me a while to discretely buy all my toys. But I eventually amassed a good collection. My electric anal toys with come hither, e-stim, tap, or thrusting action make me have wild prostate orgasms. Once I put it inside me and turn it on, I become a different person. It's pure voodoo!

I like to be on my side and curl my legs so I'm in a ball with my cock pressed back between my thighs. It can sometimes take me a while to get relaxed and situated. I need to move it around until I find the right combination of physical position and pelvic floor contractions to hold it in place. It makes me feel like an opossum giving birth in reverse.

After settling in, I let the prostate massager do most of the work. I prefer any low vibration settings with no pattern and any of the finger-like motion speeds. I get on my back and raise my legs up the wall or enjoy straddling a chair (with no arms), using a pillow to hold the toy in place, so I can rock forward until it rubs my prostate right. I feel an electric current run from the prostate up to the penis head/tip. Usually, precum follows and waves of continuous pleasure take over throughout my body. Sometimes I convulse or tense up, moan, or cry in rapture. It gets emotional for me for some reason. These waves run for a while, then stop. I chase these waves until it feels like I need to pee. That's when the good stuff follows (or flows)!

My only challenge is that the battery on my toy might run out, so I keep a few toys close for backup. I can have multiple long waves of pleasure without ejaculating. When I do feel like cumming, I release the muscle that prevents me from peeing, but I clench my ass muscle and lightly flex the muscle at the tip of my penis. I relax before fully bearing down on my ass muscle contraction as if I am strangling the toy. If I get it on just the right spot, it sends me over the edge while I pulse my tip. This continuous penile orgasm brings almost unbearable pleasure, and it lasts so long! It is so unbelievably intense, almost like electricity filling my whole body. I'm surprised I don't pee all over the floor when this sensation comes. Sometimes, I gently tap and rub the head of my cock where the pleasure is radiating most. This brings more waves of pleasure to my body. I plan to keep working on this technique, trying some different toys and positions.

I just never thought I was ever going to have anal orgasms when I first started. There's not much out there to explain things. I was trying for so long that I almost quit. Now, I look forward to doing this all the time and getting better at it."

—Jefferson

Take Me to the Afterlife

"When I ride a dildo, my target is simple. I wait until eventually it hits my prostate causing a peeing sensation. Usually, after this, pee or precum comes out of my happy cock. It is the same for a girl when her G-Spot gets hit or stimulated indirectly through anal sex. Some women squirt or at least feel like peeing. But many are too scared to let the feeling grow.

When women squirt, usually it is mostly pee. This, of course, depends on the bladder level. But generally, it smells musty and a lot like pee. As for men, it is a combination of other things like cum, prostatic fluid, and pee.

I am not afraid to let it spray! This is my favorite part of anal. That pleasurable feeling builds from riding a dildo and the precum starts leaking. As the prostate pounding continues, I can feel a tingling cumming sensation in the ass forming that spreads throughout my body. I like edging my anal orgasms, especially when I feel the strong anal contractions build. I try to make them last as long as I can. Sometimes I stop for few seconds, then start again. As they become more and more intense, I can't hold them back anymore. My cock loses control and starts squirting more precum and prostatic fluid. Eventually, cum is shooting everywhere. It's the natural order for me. And this is where my greatest orgasm begins. It's the perfect feeling of having a prostate orgasm and penile release. It feels like they go on forever.

During a good session, I find myself covered in precum and prostate juice. It's one of the most rewarding feelings of playing with your prostate. Afterward, I am dead tired and shaking from the overwhelming pleasure. But an hour later, I feel like I didn't even cum and need more. I can do these sessions 3 times in one day. I'm just a shell afterward: an assgasmed zombie for the rest of the day."

—Carter

Curiosity Killed the Pussycat

"My husband finally let me play with his sex machine.

He always did his butt stuff alone and I thought it was cute. I was curious why he loved it so much. Now I understand . . .

It started with a few drinks one weekend. We chatted about having an ultra-sex marathon. I asked, "Could I Dom you tonight?" Sheepishly, he smiled and agreed. He is usually the dominatrix, and I am the sub. Every once and while, he lets me tie him up and go to town on him, "Tame the stallion time", as he calls it in a Sylvester Stallone voice.

This time I requested we use his sex machine on him. Like a carnie at a Catholic school carnival operating a scary ride, I wanted to see the fear in his face as I controlled it. But most of all, I wanted to see how much pleasure he took from this "mechanoid mistress" of his.

I had an idea for the setup. I pulled our couches together, creating a channel between them. We safely covered them with towels and pushed the two couches back-to-back against the wall. I was able to slide the sex machine between this area and told him to sit on top. I angled his legs straight so it was like he was sitting in the street with his feet up on the curb, leaning against a wall. The wall was his headboard, and the machine pointed directly over his ass like a nuclear missile ready to launch. Watching this manly carpenter with his hands tied behind his back while blindfolded got my pussy wetter than an Atlanta waterpark in June. I took a few minutes to figure out the speeds and then I armed it with a toy from his collection: a knotted and smooth silicone shaft poked a few millimeters into his hole.

As if a professional, the layout on the coffee table had

my lube, a feather, whips, shock toys and vibrators ready for action. For the first 30 minutes, I went really slow and tortured his senses. The 9" toy's head would slide in and out deeply while he winced with pleasure. I took the feather and tickled the areas I had mapped from years of knowing him. I was surprised when he started to make ropes of precum and the dildo lathered with white ass foam so quickly. Much like a woman, he was getting wetter and wetter from our playtime. I too was dripping wet through my panties—I couldn't shake the thought of what was about to unfold for him, and it hit me hard—his ecstasy was in my hands.

Impulsively, I had to deepthroat his cock, thinking it would help me focus. Funny thing, I was the one beginning to lose control from all the arousal. It's the ultimate irony of being a Dom sometimes. As I wrestled with dizziness, I could feel him dry cumming from anal around my lips. Worried he might explode in my mouth, I stopped sucking and turned up the speed. His dildo danced back and forth more aggressively, giving him wave after wave of dry orgasms. I suddenly didn't know what to do next. It was so erotic that I was paralyzed in pleasure, feeling his orgasms sympathetically rush through me. "Keep going, I'm so close!" he yelled.

I grabbed the vibrating wand and placed it on his balls and taint. I really wanted him to suffer and beg for his creamy release. The vibrating toy made him moan and I had to gag him with a scarf so I could better concentrate. Like an artist finding her groove, I turned up the speed on my wand and his fuck toy and watched the dildo thrash his tight hole. I lightly stroked the wand across every trigger spot on his body and used my shocker whip at the same time on his dick. In less than a minute, he had a string of violent orgasms and was squirting milky streams of fluid from his cock. As his body trembled in recovery, I continued to rub and finger myself until I came, putting my fingers in his mouth so he could taste it.

I'm not going to lie, I did this to him for over two hours and lost count how many times he came from anal. After each refractory period, I just kept reapplying lube to his dildo like a water girl at a sporting match, teasing his cock ever so slightly so he would edge and be driven to madness. He was tied up and so helpless. When I was adequately satisfied with my work and his ass couldn't take anymore, I slowed down the speed of his sex machine and I climbed on top of him. I rode him until we both quickly came together.

I want to say our sex life had better moments after this experience. And there is, and always will be, incredible sex. But this night is something that I secretly fantasize about and realize it will be impossible to recreate. It was the best sex of my life!"

—Jill

Milk Marks the Spot

"I've been giving milking massages to men for years. In my milking experience, I've learned many things.

First, I start by gently stimulating the outer areas, teasing to build anticipation. After a few minutes, I move to the entrance, gradually working my way up to the prostate. Slow insertions help the anus relax. Inside, on the rectal wall, I finger to apply light pressure to the prostate, gradually increasing intensity over time. I massage it with the same gentle touch you would use on your testicles, alternating with soft tapping and light tickles for varied sensations.

They say the prostate gland is nut-shaped. I think it resembles the head of your cock and its glans; but flipped upside down. This is a good way to think about it when stimulating it. Imagine it like your frenulum and lips of the penis. Each of these areas has different sensations and can be stimulated with different micro-techniques.

The prostate lobes of your gland (the sides of your prostate) are where all the yummy juices get stored, and this is where all the prostate fluids build during arousal. Think of it like popping a pimple. I rub gently on the sides of the prostate lobes at first to get its juices flowing. It helps to arouse the gland, and makes the cock grow harder and throb. As I do this for a while, I increase the pressure and get deeper into the massage the way a masseuse does to your back and shoulders. Be creative with whatever toy or finger you use. If you do it correctly, they will want to be massaged with more pressure. A prostate needs to be milked and it loves this feeling.

As the cock gets more erect and starts to throb uncontrollably, I do get near it or touch it. The prostate pleasure can sometimes be faint for them at first and they need to concentrate on it without their cock being involved. Not long into a session, they start to drip a little cum. This is my favorite part to watch. Now, I can work the gland more confidently and milk it. I like to grip the gland between my index and middle finger and squeeze it between both fingers. I inch my fingers up as well and make various combinations of strokes, circles, and come hither movements. I focus on the sides and top of the prostate, imagining guiding the fluids toward the center of the gland. The goal is to get it engorged and hard.

This process can last 10-20 minutes or 1 hour. It depends on their stamina, sexual energy, and age. When a healthy gland is aroused, you can squeeze lots of fluid. I usually put a small container comfortably under their penis head to catch it. Many of them enjoy drinking their milk and believe it revitalizes their sexual energy quicker after orgasm.

The next area to massage is the seminal vesicles. They work together with other parts of the reproductive system. These vesicles and ampullae (sperm repositories) are what pushes ejaculate out of the penis. Knowing this helps us understand the importance and phases of milking, drainage, and orgasm.

Once the prostate gland is completely depleted of liquid, I then start to milk the seminal vesicles. These lie above the prostate gland and are harder to reach. A seminal vesicle massage gets deep, and it is a strange feeling for most since it can produce many types of emotions. If the person is aroused, it can also lead to instant orgasm. So it is important to milk these glands only when the prostate gland has been milked empty. Remember, it takes time to become engorged and hard again.

The best way to do it to yourself is to use two fingers, index and middle, together. When the fingertips go beyond the prostate gland, they can reach the seminal vesicles. There are two bulges you can feel here that start from the prostate gland and spread sideways, more deeply. The touch should start from the top and move toward the prostate gland. A light touch is needed to squeeze the fluids of seminal vesicles and draw them into the urethra. This will create thick drops of seminal fluid. That is when you know you are touching the seminal vesicles. After a stream spills out, really start to milk these glands with more force. Seminal vesicles can be drained in just a few minutes, way faster than from the prostate gland. This should produce at least half of the seminal fluid contained in a natural, penile ejaculation. From all the anal stimulation, you might also release some fluid from the Cowper's glands (precum), as well in your cum container. You can milk about two-thirds of a normal ejaculation overall without causing a full, penile orgasm if you do it correctly.

The key is to avoid triggering the penis to cum. This is the most important part of milking. It will make the final penile ejaculation more massive and intense. When someone is aroused, the glands fill with their fluids. They will be filled quickly again. This is because the testicles haven't released their sperm, they are still aroused and engorged. These are the most important glands in the male reproductive system. Milking tricks the body into thinking the internal glands haven't been emptied, so they keep working, producing more sperm and testosterone. This feedback loop in our brain continues to create the need for the body to secrete juices. It is only after an orgasm that the brain shuts off the arousal of the testicles and internal glands. Milking is all about tricking the body and mind into being a never-ending juice producing pleasure factory. We do this to cows, why not do it to ourselves and others."

—Coco

Finally!

"It took me four years trying to cum hands-free. I did everything out there. My first anal dildo finally did it. I'm so proud of myself and cried the first time it happened. And it wasn't one orgasm. I came several times. I looked down and cum and streams of fluids poured out of my pulsating cock. The harder I rode it, the more came out.

Even before this joyous day, I've always loved anal play sessions in my room. I started using a mirror, just getting into the mood and losing myself in fantasies. What helped me cum hands-free was using a large portrait-size mirror underneath me while my dildo was suctioned to it on the floor. Watching my cock flop around and seeing my hole take it is heavenly. I had my porn on the LCD projector wall and rode it furiously, up and down while clenching my ass and squeezing my left nipple. I felt like a girl wanting to milk a cock inside her. Suddenly, I lost control and felt that feeling I get when I'm about to cum from stroking it. I just kept telling myself, *You are going to cum from getting your ass fucked!* The harder I went, the closer I was getting. The more I told myself these things, the faster the feeling of unloading grew—until I just surrendered to the wave that came over me. I cried in blissful ecstasy. This was the most incredible feeling of my life. I started again and repeated this until I was unable to cum anymore.

I finished my session by using my hand and stroking. When I came from my cock, there was nothing left. Just a few little drops of clear cum. I was weeping and shaking. And I wanted to yell out the window to the world telling everyone about it. I'm already thinking how I can't wait to do this every day from now on. I'm a straight married man, but I'm wondering what it would feel like to ride a real dick. I'd probably cum in seconds. I can't wait for my wife to peg me. She's going to love making me have these types of orgasms. It will change our sex life and make things even more fun than ever, now that the roles are reversed."

—Blake

Doing Nothing Gets Me Off

"My best orgasms start with relaxation. Sometimes I take a CBD gummy. I listen to binaural beats or meditation sounds, light some candles, do some breathing techniques, or take a long shower. Once I'm totally relaxed, I keep that deep, slow-flow breathing from my diaphragm going as long as possible. I make all of my movements intentional, from arranging a towel on the bed, to getting a toy out, etc. I don't let any external or busy thoughts in this space. This is my time, and I guard it like a pit bull in a junkyard.

As soon as my Aneros goes into my ass, I close my eyes and become as still as possible. I call this the "do nothing" technique. The only thing I actually do is tune into the subtle sensations of my body, letting my fantasies take over the mood. I imagine the videos I've seen of people cumming from anal. I think about all my sex toys that I can use. I think about my partner sucking me—I let every fantasy unfold in my mind as the intense arousal and pleasure build. As this happens, my prostate starts to swell, and the prostate massager begins its locomotion.

When I finally plateau a bit, I begin my A-Muscle flexes and let the contractions pucker and pulse my hole. Continuing still and as relaxed as possible, I only flex my kegel very lightly. It's important that I let the light tingles build. I search for the perfect spot of pleasure as I hold for 3-5 seconds; then I release and let the involuntary contractions begin to come in waves. My timing is everything. It took me a while to find the right rhythms to follow, knowing to increase my squeeze, hold longer, keep my breathing consistent. I used to get too overwhelmed or sensitive and "fall off the horse". But after all my Mindgasm practice and daily kegels, I was able to find the best techniques that work for me. What also helps is not playing with my other penetrative toys, and not cumming for at least 7 days. This build-up absolutely tunes me up for anal play and gets me into anal orgasm territory easier. This brings harder P-Waves, which lead to anal orgasms and Super-Os. The more I breathe deeply and avoid holding my breath, the more mini-orgasms I have. I imagine going up a mountain and keeping the momentum upward. I keep the pleasure from leaving and use waves of pleasure as tires to get me to the top.

I used to only use dildos and vibrators to have anal orgasms. But I prefer "doing nothing" with my Aneros toy now. Less is more."

—Ray

MotivatiANAL Speaker

"I'm a big fan of prostate orgasms and have been doing it 3-5 times per week for around 15+ years. For me, the ultimate feeling is to have a prostate orgasm and a penis orgasm at the same time. I don't have them often. I wish I did because that combination always lights up the deepest feelings inside me. It feels like electricity shooting through my body. They are longer than my regular orgasms. I can have 30 in a row with no need to rest between orgasms.

Prostate orgasms make it impossible for me to be quiet and sit still. Maybe it's because I hold my breath for so long during the big ones. It feels like I was freediving 100 meters deep for 5 minutes. It feels like I ran a marathon. It feels like I took MDMA. It's such a rush, and I encourage other guys to learn how to have these types of orgasms since they are life changing. I'm not embarrassed at all to speak up about prostate play.

In my practice, I also like bigger toys now. I've moved up sizes to the largest plugs and dildos. I use some poppers to relax a bit when I do this. At first, I was surprised to be able to fit the largest toys in my ass. I learned to just ride them until I start to shake and these incredible pulsating waves radiate through my body.

Initially, it posed a challenge due to the thickness. But, with persistence, I worked on thrusting until I could successfully insert it. Gradually, over about 30 minutes, I experimented with various positions—bending over, doggy, sitting on it, and more. Eventually, it began to penetrate a bit deeper; and at that point, I lost control. I held it against my most sensitive area for roughly 20 seconds, exerting pressure, until suddenly my eyes rolled back, my knees weakened, and I nearly collapsed under the overwhelming sensations.

For the next several minutes, I continued until I reached orgasm. It marked the most intense feeling I'd ever encountered. I couldn't help but moan uncontrollably, gripping the dildo and experiencing a sensation of weightlessness. It was an orgasm unlike any I'd ever experienced before. Even after it was over, my legs continued to vibrate. And it's different from the shallower anal orgasms I grew accustomed to in the beginning of my prostate orgasm days. But don't get me wrong—all types of anal orgasms are fun!

I've become a motivational speaker to other guys. Like I said, I'm not scared to talk about it. Most guys want to listen and are curious. I just tell them the basics, that your mindset is important. Believe in yourself and don't be thinking of random stuff. Don't focus only on porn. It can help prime you, but it's not going to get you far. Don't chase the orgasm. Let it come to you. Don't cum the day before. Just relax and enjoy the feeling, like getting a massage or acupuncture.

I really believe it gets easier when you find your technique. For me, I just take the toy inside and do nothing for a few minutes, until it feels comfortable. Then I adjust my hips as needed until I find the position that warms up my prostate. When it starts feeling really good, I don't clench down. Instead, I open up like a flower, arch back a little, relax and embrace that feeling.

I love when it starts building up inside and I have some involuntary contractions. That means I'm close. I usually like to go stronger, not faster at this point. And yes, it feels like I need to pee; but when I'm doing things right it goes away, and I get some cum leaking.

Some men say they can be soft, with no erection during this phase. I'm either super hard or half-hard most of the time. I recommend that if you get soft, play with your dick a little, get hard again, then stop jerking off and go back to anal. I don't like to be flaccid. I like when it feels as if I'm cumming from my tip when a big anal orgasm hits. I think about it like my cock is a thermometer and I want the cum at about 90 degrees (80% up my urethra) when I am doing anal. This feels the best!

Just talking about this stuff is a trigger. It makes me want to play with my ass in a van down by the river."

—Tommy

The Road to Anal is Paved with Good Insertions

"If I softly rock on my suction toy, I get a buildup of feelings where my whole body becomes heavy and tingles. It hits the deepest part of my soul. It's like I have this dome-shaped sensitive muscle in my anal canal that swallows the head of the dildo while throbbing on it and getting a lot of pleasure from it. I submit to that creature within me.

I learned to surrender to that feeling and forget about ejaculations altogether, or any thought about the feelings of a penile orgasm. Only then was I able to find that next level of orgasm, which is multiple and unlimited and much stronger and more satisfying. I found new pleasures and different forms of orgasm I never knew existed. So much of it was realizing that my ability to get prostate orgasms quickly or slowly is largely due to my mental state. You have to relax, enjoy what you're doing, and take your time. Don't pressure yourself to cum. Just have fun. Enjoy the feeling of being filled and ride the waves of pleasure.

I was lucky when I started prostate exploration. I succeeded somewhat quicker than most. It took me a few weeks of experimenting to get prostate orgasms on demand. It took only a few days to learn to have multiple P-Waves. I felt my first one after 20 minutes of playing my first time with penetrating my ass. I guess you could say I'm an outlier from what I read online and hear from others. I didn't even use porn or poppers when I started.

But for years I'd always been into anal with partners and was curious about it happening to me. Exploring my dirty ass and hidden prostate held no mysteries for me. I also had zero shame or fear of seeking this pleasure.

I think a lot of anal newbies just give up too easily. They might get uncomfortable with it or sickened by the mess. They might be dealing with shame or homophobia. All of those things will slow down your learning. This kills arousal—and arousal is the fuel for your anal pleasure. Without it, you are just as useful as a proctologist sticking his finger up your ass in a sterilized exam room. Not fun!

Also, the terms "fail" and "succeed" need to be thrown out when talking about a prostate play session. If your prostate session was pleasurable even for a few seconds, that's good! Even for me, there are times when my anal play doesn't go well, and there is shit everywhere. It doesn't stop me from trying later, or tomorrow! Not all prostate orgasms are mind-blowing moments. This is important to realize, especially if you are expecting to have explosive results every time, without exception.

The mental part of anal is the primary reason people struggle with prostate play. And even if they can overcome their stereotyped conditioning, they might still struggle with technique. You will have to find the right toy (or finger), angle, depth, speed, and so on. There's a lot of variables and you have to use your own scientific method to figure it out.

The good news is that I've been doing anal play for over five years, and for me it just keeps getting better and better. Happy trails!"

—Jan

Method Man

"After a year of trying different things, I finally experienced my first dry anal orgasm. Now I can consistently achieve Super-Os at least once a week. This journey led me through some challenges and frustrating moments. But in the end, I figured out how to use various toys to understand my body better and reach orgasm without touching my penis.

First, let me be clear that what worked for me might not be the same for everyone. You can't just read things others did and expect the same results. While some tips I found were helpful, others actually made things more difficult. I needed to not be so rigid when I was starting out, thinking someone in particular was going to be my savior and mentor. It's important to consider different advice, but don't treat any of it as a strict rule for achieving a Super-O. Based on my experience, if you're similar to me, you might see results in as little as a few weeks by trying some of the methods that I suggest here.

Toys matter. I own different types of toys (vibrating, thrusting, e-stim, Aneros). Over time, I've managed to achieve orgasm with most of them (I do, however, have a duffle bag of dildos that just don't work for me anymore). The turning point came when I bought a collection of Aneros toys. I can't stress enough how much I recommend these products. I wish I had tried them sooner. While I always enjoyed the feeling of fullness of larger toys, I had no idea these smaller ones were so powerful. I mistakenly thought that Aneros products were mainly for advanced users or "weirdos", but I was proven wrong.

Getting the Aneros was a game-changer. I had tried everything, starting with dildos, exploring different angles and speeds. I'd spend hours, but I couldn't quite reach that peak to get over the hump to reach an anal orgasm. I finally discovered it's more about amplifying the sensations into waves of pleasure that become so good you have no choice but to orgasm.

Part of my challenge was a mental barrier. I psyched myself out and tried too hard to climax. But a bigger challenge was the need for breaks. Sometimes, you need to just stop and rest. Take a bathroom break, drink water . . . let the soreness and fatigue pass. The larger toys led to having fewer sessions due to more discomfort, preparation, cleanup, and difficulty taking breaks. While you can experience incredible sensations with all sorts of toys, I strongly recommend trying an Aneros in between your experimentation with vibrators and dildos.

The Aneros is a psychological toy. One key aspect of achieving a Super-O is being relaxed—not just in your muscles, but mentally. It's about focusing solely on the sensations you're feeling. You want to eliminate any distracting feelings, like the urge to pee or discomfort in your rectum from not enough lube. The Aneros is so small that it causes minimal discomfort during insertion, allowing for longer and more frequent use while staying relaxed. You just have to concentrate on the pleasure. It presses against your prostate just right and does all the work for you.

Plus, taking breaks is easy with it. You can simply get up and move around without removing the toy, although it's effortless to remove if you choose to. It can still work when you are walking around the house. This might not seem like a big deal, but the fact that using the Aneros doesn't disrupt the session as much, leads to more frequent and heightened pleasure.

In short, I had to change my approach to prostate play. This idea comes up a lot when people talk about achieving a Super-O. But I don't see it as rewiring. I view it more as training your mind to pay attention to the neglected nerves pathways in your ass. It's about letting the orgasms come to you when you are ready. A regular penile orgasm builds up the pleasure until your muscles contract for climax. During those moments, it's natural to speed up, aiming for a sensation that's a bit like pushing, as if we're sprinting toward a finish line. However, this approach won't work for a Super-O. You need to let it come to you and go with the pleasure, rather than chasing it faster and faster. Instead of trying to control it, a prostate orgasm arrives when all the elements are in place (breathing, clenching, attention to energy). Slowing down can often build more pleasure than speeding up or intensifying it. You might have come across advice that says you shouldn't focus on reaching orgasm. It is not your goal to chase the orgasm. You can definitely begin a session with the goal of achieving orgasm, there's no harm in that. But don't hold on to the outcome. Learn to train your mind and body to orgasm in a different way.

For me the pelvic floor muscles work with the Aneros subconsciously; it's similar to how we don't actively think about chewing and swallowing all that much.

Take small steps when you start out. It's all rewiring and dialing in your pelvic floor muscles. Think of it like learning to ride a bike with training wheels. In these sessions, the goal is to become accustomed to how the Aneros moves with your pelvic muscles. In my initial sessions with the Aneros, I focused on stimulating all the areas of my anus, rather than just hitting the prostate. I spent a few hours lying down with my eyes closed, or watching some porn to get used to the sensations. These sessions always ended with intense pleasure, and I eventually learned how to have dry orgasms. These early sessions were all about strengthening my pelvic muscles and adapting to the toy's capability.

I now have a routine for Super-Os that is simple. I lube up my Aneros and slowly touch myself everywhere while becoming aware of every sense and feeling. I start my kegel contractions, squeezing and holding. I like to count to 40 then relax, squeeze and hold for a 60 count and relax, increasing and holding an extra 20 seconds for each one; I grip my pelvic floor muscles slightly harder, increasing each set.

I like to visualize the toy pressing on my prostate and imagine it squeezing my prostate juice out of me. After about 10 rounds of squeezing, I release the last one as slowly as I can. This sends contractions making me shake and quiver. The key is slow, deep breaths. As the waves of muscle contractions around my prostate increase. This is when I let my body take control. Sometimes I start pulsating squeezing or reverse kegel, I just follow and focus on the center of pleasure. Eventually, the floodgates open. I leak and the contractions in my penis and around my sphincter send me into total bliss.

I don't overwhelm myself by trying to do too much at once. I search for the feeling of an impending orgasm and let it arrive in bands of waves. When I first started out, it was important to try and maintain this pace and hone in on the sensations I was getting and build from there. If you're constantly changing pace, positions, or switching rhythms, it's going to throw things off and get in the way of your orgasm.

Most importantly, the brain is the largest sex organ, and you need to train it just as much as your ass. Otherwise, it will be much harder to progress to Super-Os. If you don't learn to control your mind, it will feel much like standing inside a bucket and attempting to lift yourself up by the handle while still inside."

—Gerzog

The Quantum Orgasm

"After years of discovering the thrill of full-body orgasms through nipple play and anal orgasms, my quest evolved: I desired to unify my entire body into a single sexual entity. Along this journey, I uncovered an essence of orgasmic unity—an intensely pleasurable and deeply satisfying sensation that resides at the core of our soul. This sensation stems more from internal energy than external physical touch. Without this essential core feeling, achieving Super-Os is not attainable. This core sensation can be thought of as the epicenter of orgasmic pleasure: my neuroplexus.

When I inhabit this zone, diverse physical sensations trigger unique and captivating orgasms. Countless layers of experience lay unlocked, often left unexplored by the majority of pleasure seekers. Even the gentlest touch in this orgasmic realm generates profound pleasure, regardless of which part of my body gets stimulated. In this state, I harmonize with everything, evoking the most profound sensations and emotions within my being. It's as if a cycle of ecstasy perpetuates itself, expanding and contracting endlessly.

The range of emotions it triggers—squirting, moaning, clenching, contorting, laughing, crying—reflects its all-encompassing power. It's an experience that unifies and satisfies, forging a connection with the universe at large. Here, labels of gender, identity, and ego dissipate, all melding into the orgasmic embrace of the zone. I become one. An atom in the universe. A drop of water in the sea."

—Shaun

The Prostate Paradox: A Doctor and Patient Perspective

TRANSCRIPT: Based on a real medical case study.

Doctor: Good afternoon, RJ. How are you doing today?

RJ: I'm doing okay, Doc. I wanted to talk to you about something that's been both fascinating and, well, a bit of a challenge.

Doctor: Of course. I'm here to help. What's going on?

RJ: A while back, I had an episode of prostatitis. To alleviate the symptoms, I tried a device called the Aneros. It's designed for prostate massage. At first, I was just experimenting with it to ease discomfort, but things took an unexpected turn.

Doctor: "Unexpected"? How so?

RJ: It worked really well for the prostatitis. The symptoms cleared up in about two months, especially since I was also taking an erectile dysfunction drug daily. But during that time, I discovered the device had another effect . . . it triggered incredibly intense orgasms. I mean, I've never experienced anything like it before.

Doctor: Can you explain what you mean by "intense"?

RJ: Well, the orgasms weren't just localized. They felt like they were happening throughout my whole body. Sometimes, I'd experience involuntary muscle contractions or even shaking. It was so enjoyable that it became addictive. I ended up using the device several times a week, but it felt like I was losing control over how often I wanted to use it.

Doctor: That's understandable. Prostate stimulation can trigger powerful responses, especially if you've never experienced it before. Then what happened?

RJ: I decided to stop using the Aneros after a couple of months. The addiction was getting to me, and it felt like I was spending too much time with it. But here's the thing—I started having these orgasms without the device. Just lying prone on a couple of pillows would trigger them. No stimulation, no touching—just a reflex response.

Doctor: That's quite unique. Did you notice any physical changes or issues during this time?

RJ: Well, sometimes I'd get secretions from the urethra during these experiences, even without ejaculation. I also had an old neck injury, and some of these orgasms caused spasms in my neck, which wasn't great.

Doctor: Have you done anything to address this?

RJ: Yes. I've been working on "unwiring" myself, as some people call it. I shifted to more traditional methods, like masturbation or intercourse, and found I could have multiple orgasms during those, up to ten before finally ejaculating. But the non-stimulatory orgasms have been hard to shake off completely. I relapse every so often.

Doctor: That's not unusual, given how the brain and body adapt to such experiences. The sensations you describe appear to involve a rewiring of your reflexes and neural pathways, something that forums and discussions around this device often mention.

RJ: Exactly. The forum I visited talked about "rewiring", and I've experienced that firsthand. While I've been able to go months without those types of orgasms, I still feel drawn to them at times. It's not as simple as just stopping.

Doctor: That's a significant step forward, though. You've already made progress by recognizing the issue and taking steps to manage it. Moving forward, we can focus on strategies to help you regain balance and control, both physically and emotionally. For instance, incorporating mindfulness techniques, or pelvic physical therapy, might help you retrain your responses.

RJ: I'd be open to trying that. Honestly, I want to enjoy intimacy without feeling like I'm losing hours to this reflexive cycle.

Doctor: That's a great goal, RJ. We'll create a plan tailored to your needs, starting with some behavioral techniques. You've already taken the first steps, and that's commendable. Let's work together to get you where you want to be.

RJ: Thanks, Doc. That sounds like a plan.

Anal Means Never Say Never Again

"For a while in my mid-twenties, there was the point in my life where I was first hearing about prostate orgasms. I had a few starter toys and was learning how to explore. My roommate James and I lived in a small two-bedroom one-bath townhouse in Lansing, Michigan. He was the first gay roommate I'd ever had. James was mostly quiet, polite, and easy to get along with.

One night I came home slightly drunk and started talking about a hookup I had. I went into some details and confessed to James that I had rubbed my cock with another guy during a threesome with a girlfriend. He listened and laughed, asking, "Did you like it?"

"It was fun," I admitted, "but I was buzzed, and it was only for a few seconds."

That same night, after our conversation, I decided to bring my prostate wand to the bathroom for my shower. In front of the door mirror, I took my clothes off and played with my cock while sliding the toy in and out of me. I was still thinking about the conversation with James and couldn't resist the urge to jerk off. I lubed up my toy some more and got down on all fours. Using the mirror, I watched the toy go in and out of me while I stroked my cock in between play. The tip of the toy in my ass and the cold lube felt good. I was getting amazing feelings playing with my dick and having the toy slide inside me. I was also getting close to cumming.

All of a sudden, the bathroom door opened. I reacted instantly, closing my legs and putting my hands over my crotch.

"Oh no! I am so sorry!" James squealed. He quickly shut the door and scurried off to his room. I was so embarrassed by what just happened. I'd forgotten to lock the door and hated myself for not being more careful.

I showered then went to my bedroom. A few minutes later, James cautiously knocked on my door. This time I was in my boxers and wearing a tee-shirt, sitting on my bed. He sat down beside me, but not too close, respecting my personal space.

James said, "I should have knocked. I thought you'd gone to bed and had no idea you were in there . . ." He kept apologizing while I looked down at the floor. "I promise I'll never tell anyone. Please believe me!" He let out a sigh. "Look, we all play with ourselves. You shouldn't even be embarrassed," he reassured me, reaching over and putting a light hand on my shoulder.

I looked up and smiled, feeling better. "I know everyone does it. But it is still embarrassing. Especially since I was doing butt stuff."

"I am really sorry," he repeated.

"It's my own fault." I shrugged. "I shoulda been more careful."

We both laughed a little to cut the tension and then there was a short silence. He looked at me and asked, "Do you always do it that way?" James must have seen me driving the toy in and out of my ass.

"Not really," I said nervously. "I mean, sometimes, when I feel like it, I guess." I stood up and started folding some clothes I'd left on my bed to avoid eye contact.

"I had no idea you were into that thing," he said, "I get it. The prostate is magical. Lots of straight guys like a finger in their butt."

I didn't know what to say. "It does feel good." I allowed a smile.

He laughed. "Don't worry. Just because you like a toy in your butt doesn't mean you're gonna turn gay."

"I know." I laughed too, in relief.

And then, something came over me. I started to get an erection. It was visible through my boxer shorts. James noticed it, too. My heart raced when I looked at him, thinking, *Maybe he can teach me about prostate orgasms. I feel I can trust him with my secret. He's always nice and he has this confiding vibe about him.*

James softly asked, "Are you getting turned on by this conversation?"

I was frozen! I couldn't believe what I was thinking. It was like he was reading my thoughts. . . . *Maybe he could fuck my ass instead of me using that dildo under my bed? I've definitely thought about a real cock a few times during my anal play. But does he want to fuck me?* I knew I'd be able to take a "live" one after all the toys and experience I gained. It almost seemed to be the next logical step. I could explore a gay fantasy I occasionally had.

"I'm just still kind of horny from playing earlier," I said to test his reaction.

He raised an eyebrow. "I could help."

Without hesitation, his hand was rubbing my crotch. Soon, a wet spot of precum formed.

I reclined on the bed and closed my eyes. James took over and made me feel comfortable. He teased me and undressed me, then turned me around and bent me over.

"Do you want to fuck around and find out what a real

cock feels like?" he asked smugly.

I moaned and pushed my ass toward him. James took off his shorts and placed the tip of his dick near my hole. He started to tickle and push into my rim. James was so thick, but I had played with a thicker toy, so I wasn't scared. As I felt the head sneak inside, my brain disconnected from my body. He pushed and it inched in using his spit as lube. It felt amazing—better than any toy I'd ever used! I could see his smiling face when I looked in the mirror.

"It's in. Are you okay?" he wanted to know.

I just moaned again and buried my face into the pillow. When I looked back again, I could see his balls hanging behind mine, crashing into me. I could feel them hit my balls and it felt perfect! His cock kept grazing my prostate. I felt every inch, vein, and pulse of his cock doing its magic. He grabbed my hips with his hands as his pace increased. It was everything I imagined and more.

"Oh yes, please, fuck me harder!" I begged. I could feel the exciting friction on my prostate. "Don't stop . . . right there!" I screamed.

He pounded me furiously and I started to feel something I'd never felt before. The friction and depth slightly hurt, but the pain was delightful. I could feel his cock directly hitting my engorged prostate—it was like a finger pressing a doorbell, buzzing repeatedly in an urgent attempt to get in.

My body automatically reacted by spreading my legs more. I felt more pressure and fluid build. My eyes were shut and rolling to the back of my skull.

James continued with long strokes. In and out, every

time he hit my button, sending shivers throughout my body. I was having several mini-orgasms. He went faster and faster, then with shorter strokes, stabbing my prostate now. He grabbed my cock and yanked it. He let go, fucked me some more, then grabbed my cock again, repeating this teasing.

Having your cock played with at the same time as getting fucked is unbelievable! I couldn't hold on much longer. James was hammering away with his monster cock. He knew I was close to exploding so he stopped stroking me. But his thick hard cock pulsating against my prostate made my whole body tense, and my abdomen tightened and retracted. I felt my ass puckering and squeezing involuntarily, along with my cock. I looked down at my cock and his balls as I finally felt the release.

I came so hard from an anal orgasm that simultaneously my cum shot up to my cheek. My body convulsed and spurt ropes of cum all over my bed. James was still fucking me but wasn't far behind. My anal contractions must've sent him over the edge and he released himself into my ass. It felt like warm lube. I could feel his balls smashed against me as his cock throbbed and shot another massive load. He let out a loud grunt and collapsed on top of me.

After a few minutes, I gradually experienced a foggy and fuzzy sensation spreading through my lower body in waves and tingling in my extremities. It felt better than the best penis orgasm I've ever had and the orgasm seemed to last forever. I had officially reached the pleasure hall of fame."

—Jules

P.S. When it was all over, I went back to where it all started and took a shower. James was resting on my bed—probably thinking back about the fantastic time we had. Halfway through, I heard the door open. It was James again. I peeked through the shower curtain and saw his glowing smile. But it quickly turned to confusion when he pulled back the curtain and saw the white ooze sliding down the wall behind me.

"What is this?" he said. "We just had great sex, and you jerked off right after?"

I smiled and assured him, "I didn't cum again—I only farted."

Forgive me—I couldn't resist! My editor told me to cut this joke, then decided it was too hilarious to remove. If the P.S. offended you or distracted from the romance, may a thousand blissful prostate orgasms make up for my indiscretion. If you laughed, high five!

THE AFTERGLOW

Overview

I say goodbye and cheer you on. We hug, maybe cry—not because it's over, but because it happened.

Congratulations on making it this far in your prostranal journey! If this was a college, I'd be standing on a graduation stage handing you a diploma (or a golden dildo trophy) and shaking your hand.

Since you invested a good amount of time in this book, and we shared intimate moments, I need to tell you something. First, I am only a coach. Not a scientist, doctor, or therapist. I have no degree or certification in this field. In fact, I want you to know that I was as uninformed as you likely were, before you read this book. But while I lacked the knowledge, that didn't stop me from discovering the secrets of prostate pleasure. Once I dedicated myself to learning and practicing, there was no stopping me from achieving my first exciting anal orgasm.

The main reason I was successful with anal orgasms is that I have this steadfast trait of desiring to learn what I do not know, and to understand it fully. I want to share this final secret with you; because along your journey, it's likely you will be faced with situations where you'll open one door and then you'll be in the dark looking for the next door to open.

In this darkness, you need to figure out the "what ifs" and constantly ask new questions. That's why I recommend setting your learning and practicing goals high with the willingness to accept occasional failure. Learn from these failures to improve, then set new, refined training goals for yourself. Repeat this process with determination. If you do this, the loop of each problem and solution will close, and you'll jump to the next one with ease.

Looking back in the rearview mirror, I realize that discovering how to have consistent anal pleasure was a fun journey—one I'd gladly take all over again. I found a new world of excitement that continues to unfold even today. My persistence and dedication paid off!

But without a doubt, it would have taken me far less time if a book like this had been available when I first started.

This book is a labor of love. I want your Prostranal journey to be quick, easy, and fun—and your story to be even better.

I understand that there is a lot of information out there. When I think about it, I wish that I had ignored some of the quasi-scientific voices in the prostate community. There will be lots of low-quality and misleading information from online forums and ad-generated articles, competing to hijack your attention. This can lead to frustration or anger. It is alright to listen to what others say (e.g., what they did, or how to do it) but just remember that everyone is different, and your own body is your best teacher. Listen to it above all others. And listen to it carefully.

I can say with confidence that you've got all the tools you'll need right here. So don't wait to get started. Dive in and make the most of them. Every technique, every practice, and every story, is an opportunity for you to explore, discover, and look within to become the expert. Try the arousal amplification techniques in this book, adapt them, tweak them, and make them your own. You're about to have the time of your life as you unlock new levels of self-awareness, and ultimately limitless pleasure. Embrace the process, keep experimenting, and trust that every effort you put in will pay off. In addition to this book, I also highly recommend that you use my online training courses and audio recordings to achieve your goal even faster.

When you feel this exhilarating, orgasmic change taking place regularly—because you will!—I'll bet you won't be able to keep it to yourself. Let that excitement ripple out. And as I did, share what you're experiencing. Together, let's amplify this movement and share the message, unleashing a wave of awareness and empowerment that ripples across the world. We can invite others to discover the same ecstasy and fulfillment, transforming how they connect with their bodies and embrace their potential for pleasure.

Let's be the spark that ignites meaningful change. In a world overflowing with anger and division, what we need now more than ever is a dose of joy and connection. Prostate play might seem like a small step, but it's a powerful way to embrace pleasure, break stigmas, and bring positivity into our lives. Sometimes, **the path to a better world starts with rediscovering the joy within ourselves**.

Happy Prostraining!

Eric Win

"The Prostate Prophet"

Want to share your prostrainer story? Take part in a research study? Sign up at **prostranal.com** to join our mailing list. You may have a chance to anonymously contribute to a future edition.

RECOMMENDED RESOURCES AND COMMUNITIES

Famous People to Follow (Sexual Wellness, Podcasts, Erotica, Relationships)

- **Dr. Justin Lehmiller** – Social psychologist, sex researcher, author of *Tell Me What You Want*.
- **Dr. David Ley** – Clinical psychologist, sex researcher, expert in sexuality.
- **Dan Savage** – Sex advice columnist, host of *Savage Lovecast*.
- **Emily Morse** – Host of *Sex with Emily* podcast, sexologist.
- **Kenneth Play** – Sex educator, performance coach, expert in pleasure techniques.
- **Caitlin V** – Certified sex coach and YouTuber specializing in sexual confidence.
- **Alley Iseman** – Sexuality and wellness educator, co-founder of *Blood, Sweat & Sex*.
- **Kathy Kay** – *Strictly Anonymous podcast where you get to listen in to the secret lives of total strangers.*
- **Cam Fraser** – *Men, Sex & Pleasure podcast with discourse around masculinity and sexuality in the mainstream,*

spiritual, Tantra and sacred sexuality communities.

- **Wendy Zukerman** – *Science Vs* takes a myth-busting approach to controversial topics and current events, with fact checking and research of the scientific literature, as well as interviewing relevant experts.
- **Jamilah Mapp and Orlando Roye** – *Shameless Sex podcast covers juicy topics on love, relationships, and sexuality.*
- **Sean Jameson** – *Bad Girl's Bible podcast interviews experts and professionals and everyone in between to teach sexual tips and techniques, as well as relationship advice.*
- **Dr. Nazanin Moali** – *Sexology podcast dives into the psychology of sex and intimacy, featuring in-depth discussions with experts, psychologists, mental health practitioners, and researchers.*
- **Alexandra Fine** – *Horny for Life podcast invites people on the show to tell their unique life journey. Topics range from sex, intimacy, drugs, music and everything in between.*
- **Kim Airs** – *Sex Chat with Kim Airs interview experts in the field of sexual health and well-being, bringing sage sex advice, as well as wisdom and humor to her show.*
- **Alicia Sinclair** – *The Plug Podcast with Alicia Sinclair is all about the butt.*
- **Romaine Patterson** – *The Dildo Whisperer lets listeners have the opportunity to ask questions, hear sex toy reviews and get insight from some of the top sexperts in the industry.*

Medical Professionals & Websites (Sexual Health, Prostate Care, Urology)

- **Dr. Paul Turek** – Urologist specializing in men's reproductive health.
- **Dr. Aaron Spitz** – Urologist, author of *The Penis Book*.
- **Dr. Rachel Rubin** – Urologist and sexual medicine specialist.
- **Dr. Lawrence Levine** – Expert in Peyronie's disease and male sexual dysfunction.
- **Dr. Andrew Goldstein** – Specializes in sexual medicine (*Goldstein Urology*).
- **Dr. Richard Glickman-Simon** – Specializes in integrative sexual health.
- **Dr. Justin Elliot** – Expert in men's sexual health, urology, and erectile function.
- **International Society for Sexual Medicine (ISSM)** – www.issm.info
- **American Urological Association (AUA)** – www.auanet.org
- **Sexual Medicine Society of North America (SMSNA)** – www.smsna.org
- **Men's Health Network** – www.menshealthnetwork.org
- **Malecare – Prostate Cancer & Men's Health Support** – www.malecare.org

LGBTQ+ Communities & Support

- **CenterLink: LGBTQ+ Community Centers** – Find local LGBTQ+ centers and support groups (www. lgbtqcenters.org)
- **Planned Parenthood: LGBTQ+ Services** – Sexual health services and information tailored to LGBTQ+ individuals (www.plannedparenthood.org)
- **GLMA: Health Professionals Advancing LGBTQ+ Equality** – LGBTQ+ affirming healthcare providers and sexual health resources (www.glma.org)
- **Forge Forward** – Resources for trans survivors of trauma and sexual health education (www. forge-forward.org)

Legends in Longevity, Biohacking & Wellness

- **Andrew Huberman, Ph.D.** – Neuroscientist, host of *Huberman Lab Podcast* (brain, performance, longevity).
- **Dr. Peter Attia** – Physician focused on longevity and optimal performance, author of *Outlive.*
- **Dr. Mark Hyman** – Functional medicine expert, focuses on longevity and biohacking.
- **David Sinclair, Ph.D.** – Harvard researcher on aging, author of *Lifespan.*
- **Ben Greenfield** – Biohacker, fitness expert, host of *Ben Greenfield Life.*
- **Tim Ferriss** – Author of *The 4-Hour Body*, expert on self-experimentation and high performance.
- **Rhonda Patrick, Ph.D.** – Longevity and nutritional biochemistry researcher.

- **Dave Asprey** – Founder of *Bulletproof*, biohacker, expert in high performance.
- **Dr. Gil Blander** – Founder of *InsideTracker*, longevity scientist.

Communities & Forums (Erotica, Sexual Exploration, Fun)

- **wiki.malegspot.com** – Comprehensive guide to prostate pleasure
- **community.aneros.com** – Prostate stimulation discussions and experiences
- **r/ProstatePlay** – Reddit community for prostate stimulation techniques
- **r/CumFromAnal** – Reddit community exploring hands-free orgasms
- **r/EroticHypnosis** – Exploring pleasure through hypnosis techniques
- **r/Aneros** – Dedicated forum for Aneros users
- **FetLife** – Social network for kink and alternative sexuality (www.fetlife.com) *(Search for prostate play groups, anal play, tantra, and related topics.)*

Where to Buy Sex Toys & Pleasure Products

- **SheVibe** – Boutique adult store with a wide selection (www.shevibe.com)
- **Betty's Toy Box** – Specializes in body-safe, high-quality sex toys (www.bettystoybox.com)
- **Hustler Online Store** – Erotic products, lingerie, and adult films (www.shophustler.com)

- **Adam & Eve** – One of the largest adult toy retailers (www.adameve.com)
- **Good Vibrations** – High-quality toys, books, and educational resources (www.goodvibes.com)

Tantra & Energy-Based Sexuality

- **Tantra Festivals & Retreats** – Global listing of tantra events (www.festivalsandretreats.com/tantra-festivals-around-the-world)
- **The New Tantra** – Modern tantra courses and guided practices (www.thenewtantra.com)
- **Sacred Sexuality Network** – Tantra-focused community and resources
- **Everyday Tantra – Monique Darling and Peter Petersen** (www.everydaytantra.com)
- **Taina Ixchel – Tantra coach** (www.power-priestess.com)

Research & Academic Papers on Men's Sexual Health

- **PubMed (NIH Database)** – Search for peer-reviewed articles (www.pubmed.ncbi.nlm.nih.gov)
- **Journal of Sexual Medicine** – Cutting-edge research on sexual health (www.academic.oup.com/jsm)
- **Harvard Medical School Men's Health Blog** – (www.health.harvard.edu)
- **Kinsey Institute** – Research on topics surrounding sex (www.kinseyinstitute.org)

Prostate Health & Pleasure Books

- **Butt, Seriously: The Definitive Guide to Anal Health, Pleasure, and Everything In Between by Dr. Andrew Goldstein**
- **The Happy Prostate: A Journey to Orgasmic Bliss by Matt Hinrichs**
- **The Ultimate Guide to Prostate Pleasure** by Charlie Glickman and Aislinn Emirzian

Understanding and Overcoming Sexual Addiction

Sexual addiction, often characterized by compulsive sexual thoughts or behaviors that disrupt daily life, is a real issue for some—but recovery is possible. It's important to be aware of this before and during your prostrainer journey. It often stems from a mix of emotional, psychological, and sometimes biological factors, like using sex as a coping mechanism for stress, trauma, or low self-esteem. Recognizing the issue is the first step, and seeking professional help can offer tools to address underlying causes and foster healthier coping strategies.

Support systems are vital for recovery. For comprehensive support, the best resource is Sex Addicts Anonymous, which offers structured recovery programs tailored to sexual addiction. Visit https://saa-recovery.

org/ for access to professional help, work-shops, and educational materials designed to guide individuals toward lasting recovery.

SOURCES AND INSPIRATIONS

This book is shaped by personal experience, research, and insights from interviews, online discussions, and articles I've read over the years on human sexuality and wellness. While specific conversations aren't cited, I appreciate the collective wisdom shared by individuals. For medical and scientific accuracy, I consulted publicly available sources like Wikipedia and health-agency articles. Special thanks to the LLM models I trained and used to refine ideas and verify information.

Visit **prostranal.com** for more information, training, and resources. Sign up for regular updates and news.

ACKNOWLEDGMENTS

Well, here we are—you're holding this book, which means I actually finished it! I'd like to say it was all smooth flying, but let's be real—there were plenty of caffeine-fueled nights, questionable online searches, and moments where I seriously considered taking up foiling in Haleiwa instead of writing an "ass book".

First, a huge shoutout to my family and friends for putting up with my endless "check out this cool paragraph" moments, sudden bursts of "I am working right now!" declarations, and the occasional existential crisis of "this is going to fail miserably".

To my wife, for patiently tolerating my marathon "research sessions" and my inevitable 8 PM crashes after staying up until 3 AM writing and editing. Beyond that, her sharp analytical feedback on the book was an invaluable contribution! I'm also thankful for my sister's readiness to read my work, offer valuable suggestions, and share a laugh with me over some of the spicier chapters.

Big thanks to my editor, Cliff, for taking on this taboo topic and guiding me safely along the way, and to Books Fluent for fearlessly diving into the world of kink without worrying about getting their editing software dirty.

To my dear friends, who still stick by my side even after discovering I wrote a book about ass play—you're the real ones. To Richard Branson, Mark Cuban, Dan Koe, Alex &

Leila Hormozi, Matt Gray, and Gary Vee—you don't know me, but your genius and content have fueled my dream ship. If this book ever makes it into your hands, just know you've been part of the launch and journey (even if only in spirit).

And finally, to my readers—whether you picked up this book out of curiosity, drunkenness, or by sheer accident, you're now part of the adventure. Thanks for being here.